Schooling Sessions: A Practical Training Log for Everyday Riding

For more serious riders tracking conditioning, schooling plans, fitness goals

The Thoughtful Rider Series
Book 2

Yvonne C Caldwell

Contents

1. Welcome Dear Rider — 1
2. How to Use book — 4
3. Training Log Symbols & Short-Hand Key — 12
4. Training Mindset for Progress (Not Pressure) — 14
5. Understanding the Purpose of Schooling Work — 17
6. Schooling Exercise Ideas — 20
7. Quick Ride Plans — 25
8. Troubleshooting Guide: When Things Don't Feel Right — 29
9. Journal Pages — 40

Chapter 1
Welcome Dear Rider

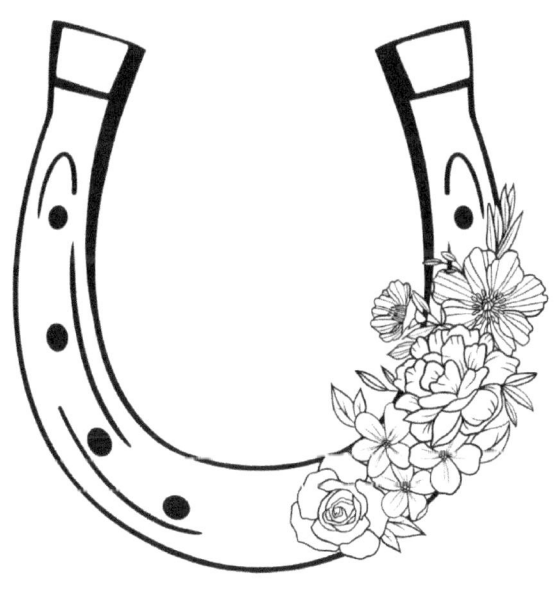

If this training log has found its way into your hands, then you are someone who rides with intention, and care about the partnership you are building with your horse. You want to improve thoughtfully, steadily, and with clarity. This book is here to support that. Schooling well takes patience.

Not dramatic breakthroughs or perfect rides, only small, consistent steps that add up over time.

This log is designed to help you notice the details and:

• Track changes in strength, balance, and relaxation

• Record the exercises and patterns that actually *work* for you and your horse

• Reflect on what helps, what hinders, and what's next

Whether you're bringing a young horse along, refining your own position, preparing for competition, or simply wanting to ride with more purpose, writing things down helps make progress **visible** — even when it feels slow.

Take your time and be curious rather than critical. Look for what improves, not what is imperfect. Your riding journey is not a race, the partnership with your horse is something you *build*, one ride at a time.

You are doing more good than you realize, your horse feels your effort.

Yvonne C Caldwell

Schooling Sessions: A Practical Training Log for Everyday Riding

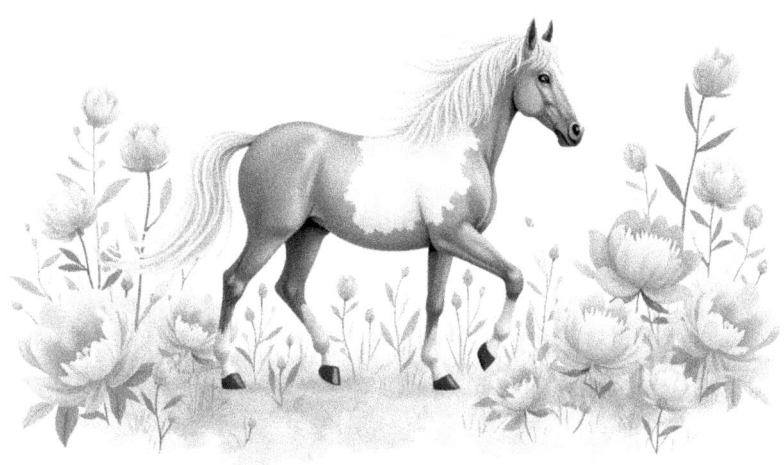

Chapter 2
How to Use book

This training log is designed to help you ride with purpose.

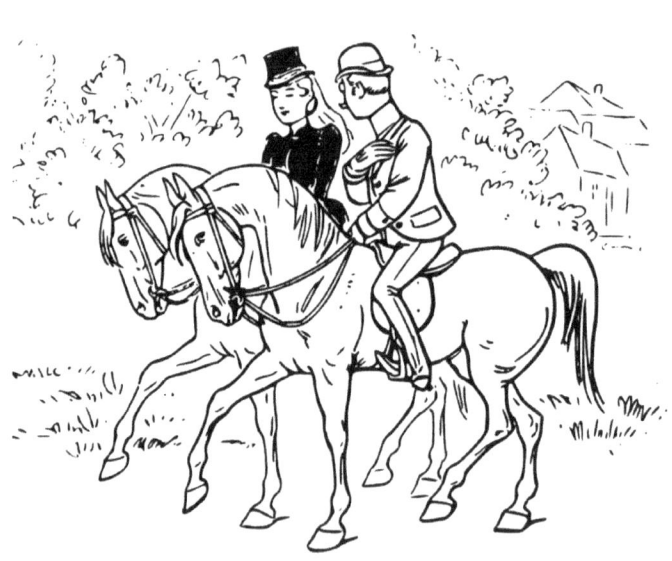

Schooling Sessions: A Practical Training Log for Everyday Riding

This training log is designed to help you ride with **purpose**. Not pressure. Not perfection. Just clear, thoughtful progress for you and your horse.

You will use this book in three main layers:

1 Weekly Planning

2 Daily Ride Reflection

3 Monthly Conditioning Review

And throughout the book, you'll find **Extra Value pages** filled with schooling exercises, quick ride plans, troubleshooting tools, and rider awareness guides to support your growth along the way.

Go slowly. Use what helps today. Return to the rest when you are ready.

1. Start Each Week with a Training Plan

The **Weekly Training Plan Page** helps you begin with direction, not guesswork.

Here, you'll:

• Choose 1–3 goals for **your horse**

• Choose 1–3 goals for **your riding**

• Map out a flexible schooling schedule (flatwork, poles, conditioning, rest days)

• Note any management needs such as farrier, bodywork, turnout changes, or saddle fit adjustments

Keep goals **small and realistic.** Consistency builds progress better than intensity. If you're unsure where to start, turn to the **Troubleshooting Guide** and ask:

What is my horse telling me they need more help with right now?

Your weekly plan is a *direction*, not a deadline. Adjust as needed — that's good horsemanship.

2. After Each Ride: Fill Out the Daily Schooling Session Log

These pages make your schooling **intentional.**

Record:

- What you focused on

- How your horse responded

- What felt like progress, even if small

- Where tension or confusion appeared

- What to carry forward into tomorrow

Small observations matter:

- *"He softened in the bend sooner today."*

- *"My shoulders stayed relaxed through transitions."*

- *"We lost balance around the corner — add shoulder-fore next ride."*

The goal is not to *review* your ride. The goal is to **understand**

your ride. This is where real progress is tracked and reinforced.

3. At the End of Each Month: Review and Reflect

Use the **Monthly Conditioning Check-In** to notice changes in:

- Strength
- Balance
- Relaxation
- Responsiveness
- Rider stability and feel

You may not see progress day-to-day. But month-to-month? You'll begin to see patterns — clear ones.

Ask yourself:

- *What has improved the most?*
- *What still needs time?*
- *Where did consistency pay off?*

This is where confidence grows: Not from perfection, from awareness.

4. Use the Extra Value Pages to Support Your Training

These pages exist to help you when you feel:

- Unsure what to work on

- Stuck in a training plateau
- Short on time
- Overwhelmed by options

Schooling Exercise Ideas

Pick 1 exercise per ride. Just one. Depth builds skill, not variety.

Quick Ride Plans (Busy Day)

Use these on days when your brain is tired, but your heart still wants to show up.

A 10-15 minute thoughtful ride is **more valuable** than an hour of distracted schooling.

Rider Body Awareness Scan

Use before mounting or mid-ride:

- Shoulders soft?
- Breathing low?
- Hips following the gait?

A relaxed rider creates a relaxed horse.

Troubleshooting Guide

When something feels *off*, flip here.

It helps you:

- Understand *why* the problem is happening
- Choose a simple, gentle correction

- Stay calm and constructive

Your horse is never "being difficult." They are showing you where balance, strength, or understanding is still developing.

Arena Pattern Sketch Pages

Use these to:

- Map exercises
- Draw jump courses
- Plan test movements
- Take notes during lessons or clinics

These become some of the most-used pages over time.

5. Go at Your Own Pace

There is **no schedule** you must follow. No expectation for how often you ride. No pressure to fill every page.

Use this log:

- For every ride

- For some rides

- For only the meaningful rides

All are correct. Progress is not linear, some weeks build strength, some weeks restore softness. Some weeks simply *keep the connection open*. Every one of those weeks matters.

A Final Thought

This book is not about riding harder.

It is about riding **smarter** - with awareness, feel, curiosity, and patience. Your horse does not need you to be perfect. They need you to be present. You are already doing the work.

This book is simply here to help you **see it more clearly.**

Schooling Sessions: A Practical Training Log for Everyday Riding

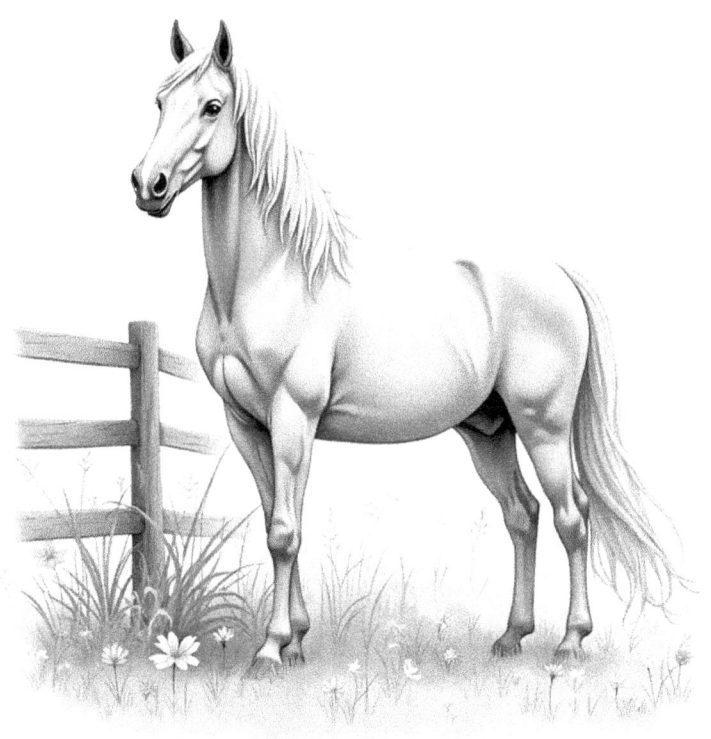

Chapter 3
Training Log Symbols & Short-Hand Key

This speeds journaling by +300%.

Symbol / Word	Meaning
↑	Increase / Improve / Add more
↓	Reduce / Soften / Slow
→	Transition / Next Step
NW	Needs Work
SW	Small Win
LDR	Long & low stretch work
SIT	Sit tall / rider posture reminder
RHYTHM	Keep tempo consistent

Schooling Sessions: A Practical Training Log for Everyday Riding

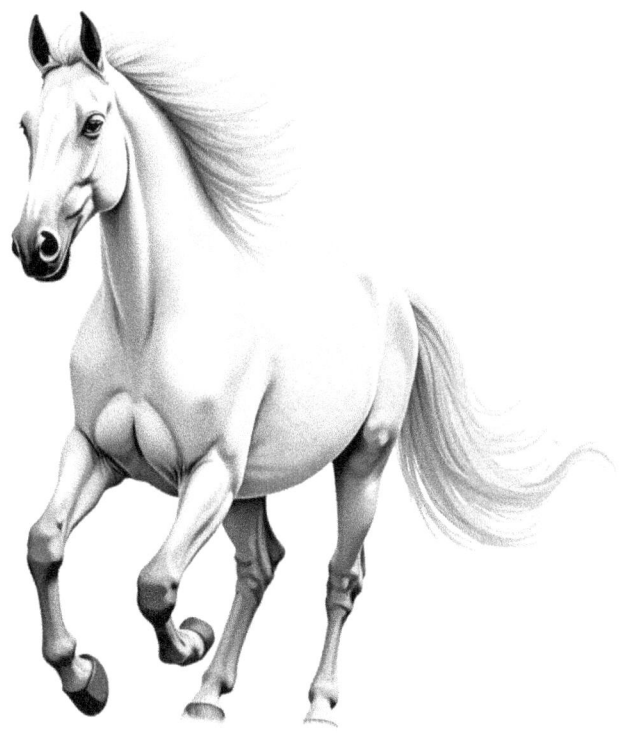

Chapter 4
Training Mindset for Progress (Not Pressure)

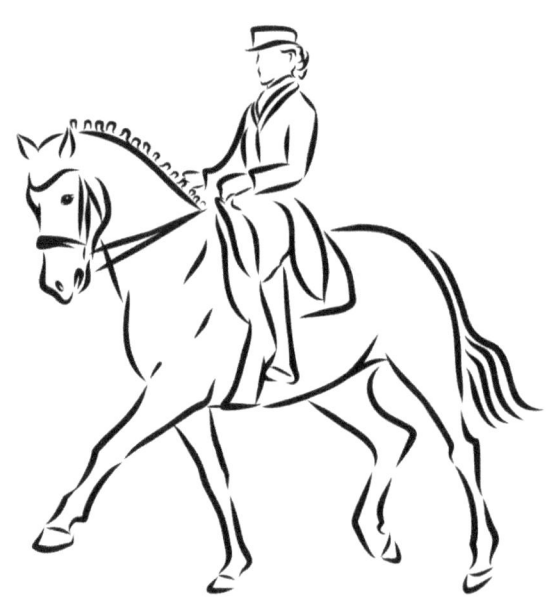

Riding is physical and technical. But training is emotional. That's why progress is rarely a straight line.

You may see:

- A good week followed by a confusing one
- A breakthrough followed by regression
- Excellent ride → unsettled ride → neutral ride → better ride again

This is *normal training curve behavior*.

The goal is not perfection.

The goal is **responsiveness + softness over time.**

When riding feels hard:

- Slow down
- Go back to rhythm
- Return to breathing
- Ride *simple* well

Simple done well is advanced.

Yvonne C Caldwell

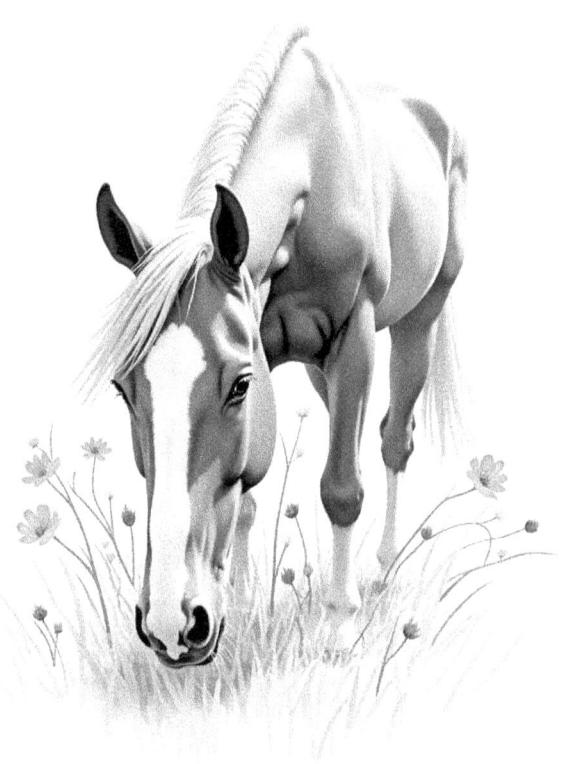

Chapter 5

Understanding the Purpose of Schooling Work

Use these when you feel stuck, bored, or unfocused

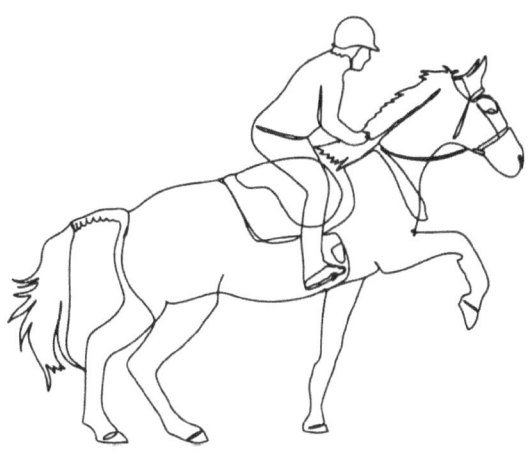

Every ride has three invisible layers:

1) Connection

How your horse and your body are communicating.

- Breath
- Contact
- Attention
- Emotional tone

2) Balance

How weight is carried and distributed.

- Straightness
- Bend
- Alignment
- Ability to shift weight gently

3) Energy

The quality of movement.

- Rhythm
- Forwardness
- Relaxation vs tension
- Adjustability within a gait

Most "problems" in training come back to one of these layers.

When unsure what to do:

→ Return to rhythm

→ Return to breath

→ Return to bend

Progress starts with soft, consistent basics.

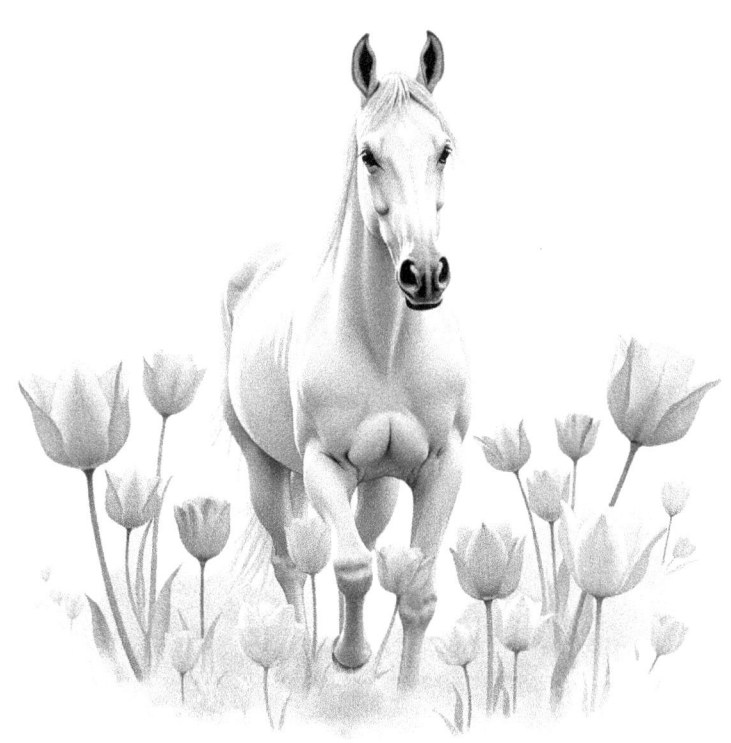

Chapter 6
Schooling Exercise Ideas

Use these when you want structure but don't want to overthink.

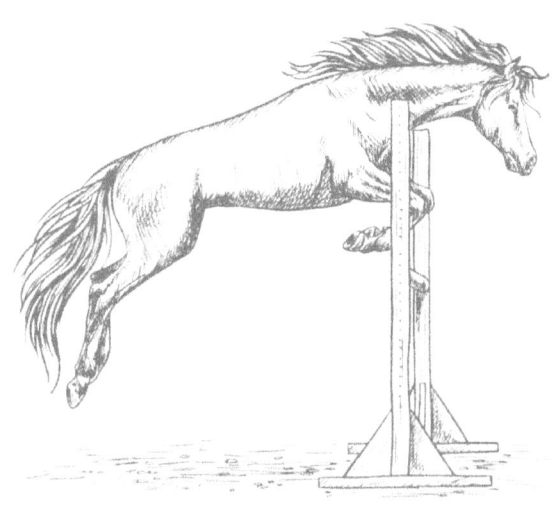

Each exercise includes:

- **Purpose**

- **What to feel for**

- **How to adjust if the horse gets tense**

SPIRAL IN → SPIRAL OUT (Walk or Trot)

How:

Ride a 20-meter circle → gradually spiral inward to ~10–12 meters → slowly allow the circle to widen back to 20 meters.

Purpose:

Improves suppleness, balance, bend, and inside-leg-to-outside-rein connection.

Feel for:

- Spine soft, not braced
- Shoulders stay tracking the circle
- Inside leg creates bend; outside rein supports shape

If tension appears:

Slow down. Make the circle bigger. Breathe.

SERPENTINE WITH GAIT CHANGES

How:

Ride a three-loop serpentine in trot. On each loop crossing, transition to walk for 3-5 steps, then back to trot.

Purpose: Improves responsiveness, focus, and balance.

Feel for:

Smooth transitions - not quick, not rushed.

If horse falls forward into transitions:

Half-halt *before* the transition, not during.

LEG-YIELD ON THE DIAGONAL

How:

Track right. At K, ride toward M, leg-yielding left.

Switch directions and repeat.

Purpose:

Straightness + response to inside leg.

Feel for:

Forward & sideways - not *only* sideways.

If horse rushes:

Slow tempo with your seat, not your hand.

CAVALLETTI FAN

How:

Place 3-5 poles in a fan shape, narrow inside distance, wider outer distance.

Purpose:

Teaches stride regulation and attention to feet.

Feel for:

Even tempo - do not "place" them with your body.

If horse gets tense:

Go back to walk over poles to reset rhythm.

LOW BOUNCE GRID

How:

X-rail → 9–10 ft → cross pole → 9–10 ft → small vertical.

Purpose:

Encourages lift, quick hind leg activity, and rider stillness.

Feel for:

You *stay quiet* - allow the horse to find the rhythm.

If horse rushes:

Add a placing pole before and after the grid.

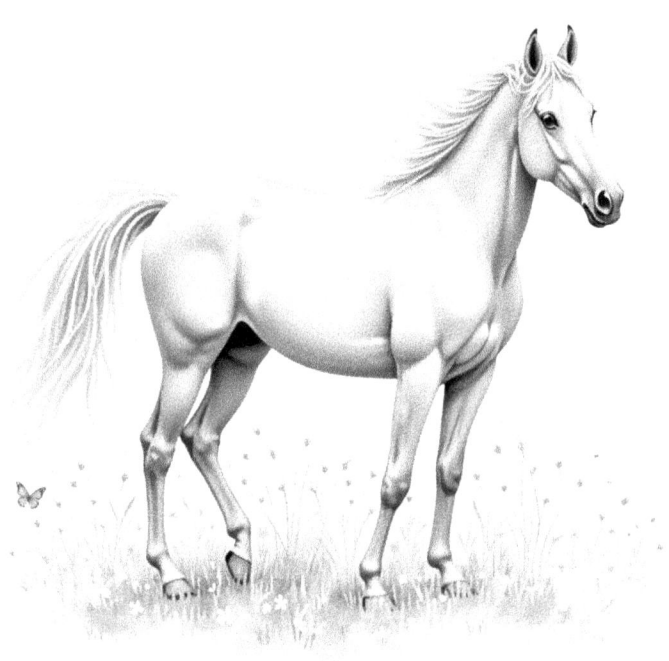

Chapter 7
Quick Ride Plans
Busy Day Schooling

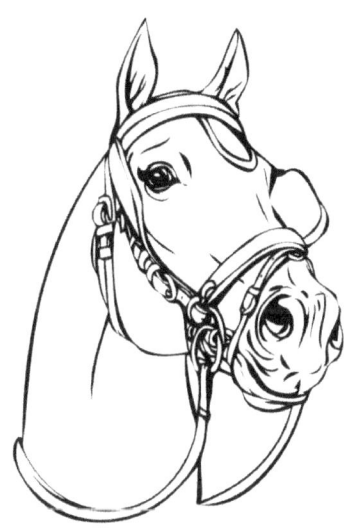

There will always be days when:

- Time is tight

- Energy is low

- Life feels heavy

- You still want to show up for your horse

These plans help make those days **worthwhile**, without pushing.

10-Minute Rhythm & Breath Reset

(The "I don't have much in me today" ride)

1 3 min: Long rein walk - big forward stepping

2 2 min: Walk → halt → walk transitions - quietly

3 3 min: Trot slow stretchy circles

4 2 min: Cool down walk

Outcome:

Calm, connected, not mentally overloaded.

15-Minute Balance & Bend Ride

1 4 min walk lateral work (leg-yield to quarter line and back)

2 6 min trot 20m → 15m → 20m circles

3 3 min stretchy trot

4 2 min cool down

Outcome:

Loosens neck + rib cage without drilling.

20-Minute Conditioning & Strength Ride

1 5 min walk hack (long rein)

2 8 min steady trot - focus on tempo consistency

3 5 min canter large loops

4 2 min cool down

Outcome:

Builds cardiovascular fitness **without** adding tension.

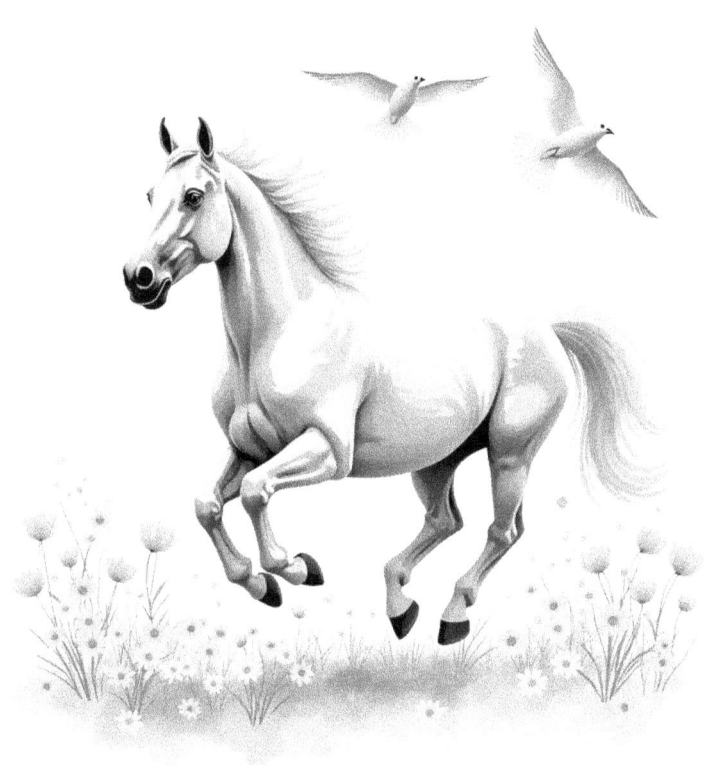

Chapter 8
Troubleshooting Guide: When Things Don't Feel Right

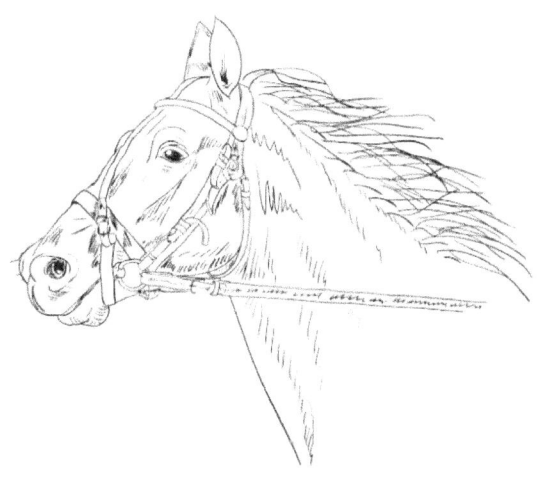

Every rider has moments where the ride feels *off*.

Not wrong, not bad, simply unclear, disconnected, or tense.

This guide helps you understand **why** something might be happening, and offers **simple, kind, and effective corrections** that support both you and your horse.

The goal is not to *fix* your horse. The goal is to **restore balance, rhythm, and communication.** Small adjustments create big change over time.

1. If Your Horse Begins Rushing

What You Feel:

Tempo speeds up, strides get choppy, horse feels "tight" in their body. Transitions may feel hurried, not thoughtful.

Likely Cause:

Tension or loss of balance.

Most horses don't rush because they are "forward" — they rush because balance has tipped.

When a horse feels like they might fall forward, the instinct is to go faster to "catch themselves."

Do NOT:

Pull back. Tighten reins. Lock shoulders. This adds more tension and confirms to the horse that something is wrong.

Try Instead:

Slow the tempo with your **seat**, not your hands.

- Deepen your breathing
- Let your hips move *with* the gait instead of bracing
- Imagine "heavy" seat bones following the stride

Add a circle:

A large, soft 20-meter circle redistributes balance without confrontation.

Goal:

Return to *relaxed forward*, not just "slower."

2. If Your Horse Feels Heavy in the Contact

What You Feel:

Weight in your hands. A feeling of being "pulled." Horse leans instead of carrying themselves.

Likely Cause:

Horse is using your hands to balance rather than engaging the hindquarters to carry weight.

This is common when a horse is weak, tense, or learning to develop topline.

Correction Principle:

Don't pull the head up. Ask the hindquarters to **step under and lift the front.**

Try:

Transitions **within** the gait.

Example:

- Trot → *slightly slower* trot → *slightly more forward* trot → repeat

- Keep rhythm steady and changes smooth

This encourages:

- Self-carriage
- Balance
- Lightness in front
- Engagement behind

Feel for:

Moments where contact feels *alive and elastic,* not heavy or rigid.

3. If Your Horse Drifts Through the Shoulder

What You Feel:

Circles get larger unintentionally. Horse leans or "falls" outward in turns. Straight lines become harder to hold.

Likely Cause:

Lack of straightness and alignment through the ribcage and shoulders. This is not about "fixing the head."

Straightness starts at the **shoulders and ribcage** — not the reins.

Correction Tool:

Shoulder-Fore

This is a mild, small version of shoulder-in — 2–3 degrees of inside flexion with shoulders slightly to the inside.

How to Ride It:

- Inside rein: ask for soft flexion

- Inside leg: supports ribcage and bend

- Outside rein + thigh: guides shoulder

The goal:

Front feet and hind feet follow the **same track.** Not more bend, more alignment. Straightness comes **from the seat and legs**, not the hands.

4. If Your Horse Feels Behind the Leg (Losing Forward)

What You Feel:

Delayed response to leg aid. Energy feels flat or sluggish. Transitions feel sticky or slow.

Likely Cause:

Horse is unsure what the leg *means* — not rebellious, not lazy. Often the rider continues *asking* instead of:

Ask → receive → release → praise

When the horse never gets to experience the release, the aid becomes meaningless.

Correction Principle:

Clarity beats pressure.

Try:

Half-halt → ask → *immediate praise and soften* EVEN if it's small. Then repeat.

The horse learns: "Forward is the answer — and forward is rewarded." Forward should feel like *willing energy,* not rushing.

Training Truth:

Soft corrections are not signs of weakness in training. They are signs of **communication and partnership.** A balanced horse becomes a willing one. A willing horse becomes a brave one.

Rider Body Awareness Scan

Your body is the horse's environment. Your breath is the rhythm your horse tunes into. Your posture, tension, and attention *shape the ride before the horse ever moves.*

This scan helps you return to **neutral, relaxed, effective riding**, especially when things get tense or confusing.

Use this **before mounting** or **anytime mid-ride** when things feel complicated.

1. Are My Shoulders Soft?

When the shoulders tighten:

- Elbows lock
- Hands stiffen
- Horse loses freedom in the neck and topline

Soften your shoulders by:

- Exhaling
- Imagining your collarbones widening
- Allowing your elbows to *float* instead of freeze

Your horse's neck and back mirror your shoulders.

2. Am I Breathing Low?

High, shallow breathing signals: "Something is wrong. Prepare to react." Low, slow breathing signals: "We're okay. Stay connected."

Try:

- Inhale through the nose for 3
- Exhale through the mouth for 4–6
- Allow belly to expand

Your horse will likely exhale in response. They are built to synchronize with you.

3. Are My Hands Following, Not Holding?

Your hands should **move with** the horse's movement, not against it.

Ask yourself:

- Are my wrists locked?
- Am I trying to "hold the frame?"
- Or am I allowing softness and release?

A hand that follows says: "Stay with me."

A hand that holds says: "Don't move."

The horse will choose softness when softness is available.

4. Can My Hips Swing Freely?

Your seat is where communication begins.

If your hips are:

- Gripping

- Bracing

- Tight

- Tipped forward or back

The horse loses access to rhythm.

Let your hips follow the stride:

- Walk: side-to-side flow

- Trot: gentle lift and return

- Canter: rolling wave-like motion

Your horse reads **your seat** as leadership.

5. Where is My Attention?

There are only two places your attention can be:

- On your horse

- On how you *think* you're doing

One leads to communication. The other leads to tension.

Shift your focus to:

- Rhythm
- Breath
- Feel
- Softness

Your horse does not want perfection. They want presence.

Body Scan Summary

Return to:

Alignment → Rhythm → Breath.

This resets:

- The nervous system
- The communication system
- The training system

This simple reset solves more problems than force ever will.

Final Note

Your horse does not improve because you demand more. Your horse improves because you create an environment where learning feels safe, steady, and clear. Your training is a conversation. Not a performance. You are doing thoughtful work. Your horse feels the difference.

Schooling Sessions: A Practical Training Log for Everyday Riding

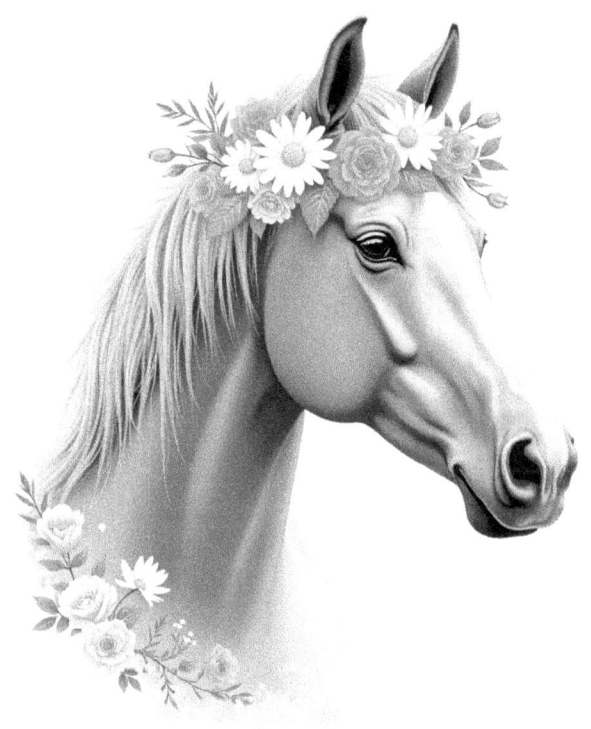

Chapter 9
Journal Pages

WEEKLY TRAINING PLAN

DAILY SCHOOLING SESSION LOG

MONTHLY CONDITIONING CHECK-IN

Weekly Training Plan

Week of: _____ *Weekly Training Plan*

This Week's Goals

Horse Focus

_____

_____

_____

Rider Focus

_____

_____

_____

Conditioning & Schooling Schedule

(Examples: long and low day, cavaletti day, hill conditioning, lunge + stretch day)

Day	Plan / Exercise Focus	Notes
Mon	_____	_____
Tue	_____	_____
Wed	_____	_____
Thu	_____	_____
Fri	_____	_____
Sat	_____	_____
	_____	_____

Primary Skill Focus This Week

(Check or circle 1–3)

- ☐ Transitions
- ☐ Rhythm & Tempo
- ☐ Straightness
- ☐ Bend / Lateral Suppleness
- ☐ Engagement Behind
- ☐ Contact & Connection
- ☐ Adjustability / Stride Control
- ☐ Rideability / Focus
- ☐ Rider Position & Balance
- ☐ Jump Form / Gridwork

Notes:

Barn & Horse Management Notes

(Farrier, chiro, saddle fitter, health changes, shoeing, turnout, etc.)

Week of: _____ # Weekly Training Plan

This Week's Goals

Horse Focus

_____

_____

_____

Rider Focus

_____

_____

_____

Conditioning & Schooling Schedule

(Examples: long and low day, cavaletti day, hill conditioning, lunge + stretch day)

Day	Plan / Exercise Focus	Notes
Mon	_____	_____
Tue	_____	_____
Wed	_____	_____
Thu	_____	_____
Fri	_____	_____
Sat	_____	_____
Sun	_____	_____

Primary Skill Focus This Week

(Check or circle 1–3)

- ☐ Transitions
- ☐ Rhythm & Tempo
- ☐ Straightness
- ☐ Bend / Lateral Suppleness
- ☐ Engagement Behind
- ☐ Contact & Connection
- ☐ Adjustability / Stride Control
- ☐ Rideability / Focus
- ☐ Rider Position & Balance
- ☐ Jump Form / Gridwork

Notes:

Barn & Horse Management Notes

(Farrier, chiro, saddle fitter, health changes, shoeing, turnout, etc.)

Week of: _____ *Weekly Training Plan*

This Week's Goals

Horse Focus

_____

_____

_____

Rider Focus

_____

_____

_____

Conditioning & Schooling Schedule

(Examples: long and low day, cavaletti day, hill conditioning, lunge + stretch day)

Day	Plan / Exercise Focus	Notes
Mon	_____	_____
Tue	_____	_____
Wed	_____	_____
Thu	_____	_____
Fri	_____	_____
Sat	_____	_____
Sun	_____	_____

Primary Skill Focus This Week

(Check or circle 1–3)

- ☐ Transitions
- ☐ Rhythm & Tempo
- ☐ Straightness
- ☐ Bend / Lateral Suppleness
- ☐ Engagement Behind
- ☐ Contact & Connection
- ☐ Adjustability / Stride Control
- ☐ Rideability / Focus
- ☐ Rider Position & Balance
- ☐ Jump Form / Gridwork

Notes:

Barn & Horse Management Notes

(Farrier, chiro, saddle fitter, health changes, shoeing, turnout, etc.)

Week of: _____ *Weekly Training Plan*

This Week's Goals

Horse Focus

_____

_____

_____

Rider Focus

_____

_____

_____

Conditioning & Schooling Schedule

(Examples: long and low day, cavaletti day, hill conditioning, lunge + stretch day)

Day	Plan / Exercise Focus	Notes
Mon	_____	_____
Tue	_____	_____
Wed	_____	_____
Thu	_____	_____
Fri	_____	_____
Sat	_____	_____
Sun	_____	_____

Primary Skill Focus This Week

(Check or circle 1–3)

- ☐ Transitions
- ☐ Rhythm & Tempo
- ☐ Straightness
- ☐ Bend / Lateral Suppleness
- ☐ Engagement Behind
- ☐ Contact & Connection
- ☐ Adjustability / Stride Control
- ☐ Rideability / Focus
- ☐ Rider Position & Balance
- ☐ Jump Form / Gridwork

Notes:

Barn & Horse Management Notes

(Farrier, chiro, saddle fitter, health changes, shoeing, turnout, etc.)

Week of: _____   *Weekly Training Plan*

This Week's Goals

Horse Focus

_____

_____

_____

Rider Focus

_____

_____

_____

Conditioning & Schooling Schedule

(Examples: long and low day, cavaletti day, hill conditioning, lunge + stretch day)

Day	Plan / Exercise Focus	Notes
Mon	_____	_____
Tue	_____	_____
Wed	_____	_____
Thu	_____	_____
Fri	_____	_____
Sat	_____	_____
Sun	_____	_____

Primary Skill Focus This Week

(Check or circle 1–3)

- ☐ Transitions
- ☐ Rhythm & Tempo
- ☐ Straightness
- ☐ Bend / Lateral Suppleness
- ☐ Engagement Behind
- ☐ Contact & Connection
- ☐ Adjustability / Stride Control
- ☐ Rideability / Focus
- ☐ Rider Position & Balance
- ☐ Jump Form / Gridwork

Notes:

Barn & Horse Management Notes

(Farrier, chiro, saddle fitter, health changes, shoeing, turnout, etc.)

Week of: _____ *Weekly Training Plan*

This Week's Goals

Horse Focus

_____

_____

_____

Rider Focus

_____

_____

_____

Conditioning & Schooling Schedule

(Examples: long and low day, cavaletti day, hill conditioning, lunge + stretch day)

Day	Plan / Exercise Focus	Notes
Mon	_____	_____
Tue	_____	_____
Wed	_____	_____
Thu	_____	_____
Fri	_____	_____
Sat	_____	_____
Sun	_____	_____

Primary Skill Focus This Week

(Check or circle 1–3)

- ☐ Transitions
- ☐ Rhythm & Tempo
- ☐ Straightness
- ☐ Bend / Lateral Suppleness
- ☐ Engagement Behind
- ☐ Contact & Connection
- ☐ Adjustability / Stride Control
- ☐ Rideability / Focus
- ☐ Rider Position & Balance
- ☐ Jump Form / Gridwork

Notes:

Barn & Horse Management Notes

(Farrier, chiro, saddle fitter, health changes, shoeing, turnout, etc.)

Week of: _____ *Weekly Training Plan*

This Week's Goals

Horse Focus

_____

_____

_____

Rider Focus

_____

_____

_____

Conditioning & Schooling Schedule

(Examples: long and low day, cavaletti day, hill conditioning, lunge + stretch day)

Day	Plan / Exercise Focus	Notes
Mon	_____	_____
Tue	_____	_____
Wed	_____	_____
Thu	_____	_____
Fri	_____	_____
Sat	_____	_____
Sun	_____	_____

Primary Skill Focus This Week

(Check or circle 1–3)

- ☐ Transitions
- ☐ Rhythm & Tempo
- ☐ Straightness
- ☐ Bend / Lateral Suppleness
- ☐ Engagement Behind
- ☐ Contact & Connection
- ☐ Adjustability / Stride Control
- ☐ Rideability / Focus
- ☐ Rider Position & Balance
- ☐ Jump Form / Gridwork

Notes:

Barn & Horse Management Notes

(Farrier, chiro, saddle fitter, health changes, shoeing, turnout, etc.)

Week of: _____ *Weekly Training Plan*

This Week's Goals

Horse Focus

_____

_____

_____

Rider Focus

_____

_____

_____

Conditioning & Schooling Schedule

(Examples: long and low day, cavaletti day, hill conditioning, lunge + stretch day)

Day	Plan / Exercise Focus	Notes
Mon	_____	_____
Tue	_____	_____
Wed	_____	_____
Thu	_____	_____
Fri	_____	_____
Sat	_____	_____
Sun	_____	_____

Primary Skill Focus This Week

(Check or circle 1–3)

- ☐ Transitions
- ☐ Rhythm & Tempo
- ☐ Straightness
- ☐ Bend / Lateral Suppleness
- ☐ Engagement Behind
- ☐ Contact & Connection
- ☐ Adjustability / Stride Control
- ☐ Rideability / Focus
- ☐ Rider Position & Balance
- ☐ Jump Form / Gridwork

Notes:

Barn & Horse Management Notes

(Farrier, chiro, saddle fitter, health changes, shoeing, turnout, etc.)

Week of: _____   *Weekly Training Plan*

This Week's Goals

Horse Focus

_____

_____

_____

Rider Focus

_____

_____

_____

Conditioning & Schooling Schedule

(Examples: long and low day, cavaletti day, hill conditioning, lunge + stretch day)

Day	Plan / Exercise Focus	Notes
Mon	_____	_____
Tue	_____	_____
Wed	_____	_____
Thu	_____	_____
Fri	_____	_____
Sat	_____	_____
Sun	_____	_____

Primary Skill Focus This Week

(Check or circle 1–3)

- ☐ Transitions
- ☐ Rhythm & Tempo
- ☐ Straightness
- ☐ Bend / Lateral Suppleness
- ☐ Engagement Behind
- ☐ Contact & Connection
- ☐ Adjustability / Stride Control
- ☐ Rideability / Focus
- ☐ Rider Position & Balance
- ☐ Jump Form / Gridwork

Notes:

Barn & Horse Management Notes

(Farrier, chiro, saddle fitter, health changes, shoeing, turnout, etc.)

Week of: _____ *Weekly Training Plan*

This Week's Goals

Horse Focus

_____

_____

_____

Rider Focus

_____

_____

_____

Conditioning & Schooling Schedule

(Examples: long and low day, cavaletti day, hill conditioning, lunge + stretch day)

Day	Plan / Exercise Focus	Notes
Mon	_____	_____
Tue	_____	_____
Wed	_____	_____
Thu	_____	_____
Fri	_____	_____
Sat	_____	_____
Sun	_____	_____

Primary Skill Focus This Week

(Check or circle 1–3)

- ☐ Transitions
- ☐ Rhythm & Tempo
- ☐ Straightness
- ☐ Bend / Lateral Suppleness
- ☐ Engagement Behind
- ☐ Contact & Connection
- ☐ Adjustability / Stride Control
- ☐ Rideability / Focus
- ☐ Rider Position & Balance
- ☐ Jump Form / Gridwork

Notes:

Barn & Horse Management Notes

(Farrier, chiro, saddle fitter, health changes, shoeing, turnout, etc.)

Week of: _____ *Weekly Training Plan*

This Week's Goals

Horse Focus

_____

_____

_____

Rider Focus

_____

_____

_____

Conditioning & Schooling Schedule

(Examples: long and low day, cavaletti day, hill conditioning, lunge + stretch day)

Day	Plan / Exercise Focus	Notes
Mon	_____	_____
Tue	_____	_____
Wed	_____	_____
Thu	_____	_____
Fri	_____	_____
Sat	_____	_____
Sun	_____	_____

Primary Skill Focus This Week

(Check or circle 1–3)

- ☐ Transitions
- ☐ Rhythm & Tempo
- ☐ Straightness
- ☐ Bend / Lateral Suppleness
- ☐ Engagement Behind
- ☐ Contact & Connection
- ☐ Adjustability / Stride Control
- ☐ Rideability / Focus
- ☐ Rider Position & Balance
- ☐ Jump Form / Gridwork

Notes:

Barn & Horse Management Notes

(Farrier, chiro, saddle fitter, health changes, shoeing, turnout, etc.)

Week of: _____ *Weekly Training Plan*

This Week's Goals

Horse Focus

_____

_____

_____

Rider Focus

_____

_____

_____

Conditioning & Schooling Schedule

(Examples: long and low day, cavaletti day, hill conditioning, lunge + stretch day)

Day	Plan / Exercise Focus	Notes
Mon	_____	_____
Tue	_____	_____
Wed	_____	_____
Thu	_____	_____
Fri	_____	_____
Sat	_____	_____
Sun	_____	_____

Primary Skill Focus This Week

(Check or circle 1–3)

- ☐ Transitions
- ☐ Rhythm & Tempo
- ☐ Straightness
- ☐ Bend / Lateral Suppleness
- ☐ Engagement Behind
- ☐ Contact & Connection
- ☐ Adjustability / Stride Control
- ☐ Rideability / Focus
- ☐ Rider Position & Balance
- ☐ Jump Form / Gridwork

Notes:

Barn & Horse Management Notes

(Farrier, chiro, saddle fitter, health changes, shoeing, turnout, etc.)

Week of: _____ *Weekly Training Plan*

This Week's Goals

Horse Focus

_____

_____

_____

Rider Focus

_____

_____

_____

Conditioning & Schooling Schedule

(Examples: long and low day, cavaletti day, hill conditioning, lunge + stretch day)

Day	Plan / Exercise Focus	Notes
Mon	_____	_____
Tue	_____	_____
Wed	_____	_____
Thu	_____	_____
Fri	_____	_____
Sat	_____	_____
Sun	_____	_____

Primary Skill Focus This Week

(Check or circle 1–3)

- ☐ Transitions
- ☐ Rhythm & Tempo
- ☐ Straightness
- ☐ Bend / Lateral Suppleness
- ☐ Engagement Behind
- ☐ Contact & Connection
- ☐ Adjustability / Stride Control
- ☐ Rideability / Focus
- ☐ Rider Position & Balance
- ☐ Jump Form / Gridwork

Notes:

Barn & Horse Management Notes

(Farrier, chiro, saddle fitter, health changes, shoeing, turnout, etc.)

Week of: _____ *Weekly Training Plan*

This Week's Goals

Horse Focus

_____

_____

_____

Rider Focus

_____

_____

_____

Conditioning & Schooling Schedule

(Examples: long and low day, cavaletti day, hill conditioning, lunge + stretch day)

Day	Plan / Exercise Focus	Notes
Mon	_____	_____
Tue	_____	_____
Wed	_____	_____
Thu	_____	_____
Fri	_____	_____
Sat	_____	_____
Sun	_____	_____

Primary Skill Focus This Week

(Check or circle 1–3)

- ☐ Transitions
- ☐ Rhythm & Tempo
- ☐ Straightness
- ☐ Bend / Lateral Suppleness
- ☐ Engagement Behind
- ☐ Contact & Connection
- ☐ Adjustability / Stride Control
- ☐ Rideability / Focus
- ☐ Rider Position & Balance
- ☐ Jump Form / Gridwork

Notes:

Barn & Horse Management Notes

(Farrier, chiro, saddle fitter, health changes, shoeing, turnout, etc.)

Week of: _____ *Weekly Training Plan*

This Week's Goals

Horse Focus

_____

_____

_____

Rider Focus

_____

_____

_____

Conditioning & Schooling Schedule

(Examples: long and low day, cavaletti day, hill conditioning, lunge + stretch day)

Day	Plan / Exercise Focus	Notes
Mon	_____	_____
Tue	_____	_____
Wed	_____	_____
Thu	_____	_____
Fri	_____	_____
Sat	_____	_____
Sun	_____	_____

Primary Skill Focus This Week

(Check or circle 1–3)

- ☐ Transitions
- ☐ Rhythm & Tempo
- ☐ Straightness
- ☐ Bend / Lateral Suppleness
- ☐ Engagement Behind
- ☐ Contact & Connection
- ☐ Adjustability / Stride Control
- ☐ Rideability / Focus
- ☐ Rider Position & Balance
- ☐ Jump Form / Gridwork

Notes:

Barn & Horse Management Notes

(Farrier, chiro, saddle fitter, health changes, shoeing, turnout, etc.)

Week of: _____ *Weekly Training Plan*

This Week's Goals

Horse Focus

_____

_____

_____

Rider Focus

_____

_____

_____

Conditioning & Schooling Schedule

(Examples: long and low day, cavaletti day, hill conditioning, lunge + stretch day)

Day	Plan / Exercise Focus	Notes
Mon	_____	_____
Tue	_____	_____
Wed	_____	_____
Thu	_____	_____
Fri	_____	_____
Sat	_____	_____
Sun	_____	_____

Primary Skill Focus This Week

(Check or circle 1–3)

- ☐ Transitions
- ☐ Rhythm & Tempo
- ☐ Straightness
- ☐ Bend / Lateral Suppleness
- ☐ Engagement Behind
- ☐ Contact & Connection
- ☐ Adjustability / Stride Control
- ☐ Rideability / Focus
- ☐ Rider Position & Balance
- ☐ Jump Form / Gridwork

Notes:

Barn & Horse Management Notes

(Farrier, chiro, saddle fitter, health changes, shoeing, turnout, etc.)

Week of: _____ *Weekly Training Plan*

This Week's Goals

Horse Focus

_____

_____

_____

Rider Focus

_____

_____

_____

Conditioning & Schooling Schedule

(Examples: long and low day, cavaletti day, hill conditioning, lunge + stretch day)

Day	Plan / Exercise Focus	Notes
Mon	_____	_____
Tue	_____	_____
Wed	_____	_____
Thu	_____	_____
Fri	_____	_____
Sat	_____	_____
	_____	_____

Primary Skill Focus This Week

(Check or circle 1–3)

- ☐ Transitions
- ☐ Rhythm & Tempo
- ☐ Straightness
- ☐ Bend / Lateral Suppleness
- ☐ Engagement Behind
- ☐ Contact & Connection
- ☐ Adjustability / Stride Control
- ☐ Rideability / Focus
- ☐ Rider Position & Balance
- ☐ Jump Form / Gridwork

Notes:

Barn & Horse Management Notes

(Farrier, chiro, saddle fitter, health changes, shoeing, turnout, etc.)

Week of: _____ # Weekly Training Plan

This Week's Goals

Horse Focus

_____

_____

_____

Rider Focus

_____

_____

_____

Conditioning & Schooling Schedule

(Examples: long and low day, cavaletti day, hill conditioning, lunge + stretch day)

Day	Plan / Exercise Focus	Notes
Mon	_____	_____
Tue	_____	_____
Wed	_____	_____
Thu	_____	_____
Fri	_____	_____
Sat	_____	_____
Sun	_____	_____

Primary Skill Focus This Week

(Check or circle 1–3)

- ☐ Transitions
- ☐ Rhythm & Tempo
- ☐ Straightness
- ☐ Bend / Lateral Suppleness
- ☐ Engagement Behind
- ☐ Contact & Connection
- ☐ Adjustability / Stride Control
- ☐ Rideability / Focus
- ☐ Rider Position & Balance
- ☐ Jump Form / Gridwork

Notes:

Barn & Horse Management Notes

(Farrier, chiro, saddle fitter, health changes, shoeing, turnout, etc.)

Week of: _____ *Weekly Training Plan*

This Week's Goals

Horse Focus

_____

_____

_____

Rider Focus

_____

_____

_____

Conditioning & Schooling Schedule

(Examples: long and low day, cavaletti day, hill conditioning, lunge + stretch day)

Day	Plan / Exercise Focus	Notes
Mon	_____	_____
Tue	_____	_____
Wed	_____	_____
Thu	_____	_____
Fri	_____	_____
Sat	_____	_____
Sun	_____	_____

Primary Skill Focus This Week

(Check or circle 1–3)

- ☐ Transitions
- ☐ Rhythm & Tempo
- ☐ Straightness
- ☐ Bend / Lateral Suppleness
- ☐ Engagement Behind
- ☐ Contact & Connection
- ☐ Adjustability / Stride Control
- ☐ Rideability / Focus
- ☐ Rider Position & Balance
- ☐ Jump Form / Gridwork

Notes:

Barn & Horse Management Notes

(Farrier, chiro, saddle fitter, health changes, shoeing, turnout, etc.)

Week of: _____ *Weekly Training Plan*

This Week's Goals

Horse Focus

_____

_____

_____

Rider Focus

_____

_____

_____

Conditioning & Schooling Schedule

(Examples: long and low day, cavaletti day, hill conditioning, lunge + stretch day)

Day	Plan / Exercise Focus	Notes
Mon	_____	_____
Tue	_____	_____
Wed	_____	_____
Thu	_____	_____
Fri	_____	_____
Sat	_____	_____
Sun	_____	_____

Primary Skill Focus This Week

(Check or circle 1–3)

- ☐ Transitions
- ☐ Rhythm & Tempo
- ☐ Straightness
- ☐ Bend / Lateral Suppleness
- ☐ Engagement Behind
- ☐ Contact & Connection
- ☐ Adjustability / Stride Control
- ☐ Rideability / Focus
- ☐ Rider Position & Balance
- ☐ Jump Form / Gridwork

Notes:

Barn & Horse Management Notes

(Farrier, chiro, saddle fitter, health changes, shoeing, turnout, etc.)

Week of: _____   *Weekly Training Plan*

This Week's Goals

Horse Focus

_____

_____

_____

Rider Focus

_____

_____

_____

Conditioning & Schooling Schedule

(Examples: long and low day, cavaletti day, hill conditioning, lunge + stretch day)

Day	Plan / Exercise Focus	Notes
Mon	_____	_____
Tue	_____	_____
Wed	_____	_____
Thu	_____	_____
Fri	_____	_____
Sat	_____	_____
Sun	_____	_____

Primary Skill Focus This Week

(Check or circle 1–3)

- ☐ Transitions
- ☐ Rhythm & Tempo
- ☐ Straightness
- ☐ Bend / Lateral Suppleness
- ☐ Engagement Behind
- ☐ Contact & Connection
- ☐ Adjustability / Stride Control
- ☐ Rideability / Focus
- ☐ Rider Position & Balance
- ☐ Jump Form / Gridwork

Notes:

Barn & Horse Management Notes

(Farrier, chiro, saddle fitter, health changes, shoeing, turnout, etc.)

Week of: _____ *Weekly Training Plan*

This Week's Goals

Horse Focus

_____

_____

_____

Rider Focus

_____

_____

_____

Conditioning & Schooling Schedule

(Examples: long and low day, cavaletti day, hill conditioning, lunge + stretch day)

Day	Plan / Exercise Focus	Notes
Mon	_____	_____
Tue	_____	_____
Wed	_____	_____
Thu	_____	_____
Fri	_____	_____
Sat	_____	_____
Sun	_____	_____

Primary Skill Focus This Week

(Check or circle 1–3)

- ☐ Transitions
- ☐ Rhythm & Tempo
- ☐ Straightness
- ☐ Bend / Lateral Suppleness
- ☐ Engagement Behind
- ☐ Contact & Connection
- ☐ Adjustability / Stride Control
- ☐ Rideability / Focus
- ☐ Rider Position & Balance
- ☐ Jump Form / Gridwork

Notes:

Barn & Horse Management Notes

(Farrier, chiro, saddle fitter, health changes, shoeing, turnout, etc.)

Week of: _____   *Weekly Training Plan*

This Week's Goals

Horse Focus

_____

_____

_____

Rider Focus

_____

_____

_____

Conditioning & Schooling Schedule

(Examples: long and low day, cavaletti day, hill conditioning, lunge + stretch day)

Day	Plan / Exercise Focus	Notes
Mon	_____	_____
Tue	_____	_____
Wed	_____	_____
Thu	_____	_____
Fri	_____	_____
Sat	_____	_____
Sun	_____	_____

Primary Skill Focus This Week

(Check or circle 1–3)

- ☐ Transitions
- ☐ Rhythm & Tempo
- ☐ Straightness
- ☐ Bend / Lateral Suppleness
- ☐ Engagement Behind
- ☐ Contact & Connection
- ☐ Adjustability / Stride Control
- ☐ Rideability / Focus
- ☐ Rider Position & Balance
- ☐ Jump Form / Gridwork

Notes:

Barn & Horse Management Notes

(Farrier, chiro, saddle fitter, health changes, shoeing, turnout, etc.)

Week of: _____ *Weekly Training Plan*

This Week's Goals

Horse Focus

_____

_____

_____

Rider Focus

_____

_____

_____

Conditioning & Schooling Schedule

(Examples: long and low day, cavaletti day, hill conditioning, lunge + stretch day)

Day	Plan / Exercise Focus	Notes
Mon	_____	_____
Tue	_____	_____
Wed	_____	_____
Thu	_____	_____
Fri	_____	_____
Sat	_____	_____
Sun	_____	_____

Primary Skill Focus This Week

(Check or circle 1–3)

- ☐ Transitions
- ☐ Rhythm & Tempo
- ☐ Straightness
- ☐ Bend / Lateral Suppleness
- ☐ Engagement Behind
- ☐ Contact & Connection
- ☐ Adjustability / Stride Control
- ☐ Rideability / Focus
- ☐ Rider Position & Balance
- ☐ Jump Form / Gridwork

Notes:

Barn & Horse Management Notes

(Farrier, chiro, saddle fitter, health changes, shoeing, turnout, etc.)

Week of: _____   *Weekly Training Plan*

This Week's Goals

Horse Focus

_____

_____

_____

Rider Focus

_____

_____

_____

Conditioning & Schooling Schedule

(Examples: long and low day, cavaletti day, hill conditioning, lunge + stretch day)

Day	Plan / Exercise Focus	Notes
Mon	_____	_____
Tue	_____	_____
Wed	_____	_____
Thu	_____	_____
Fri	_____	_____
Sat	_____	_____
Sun	_____	_____

Primary Skill Focus This Week

(Check or circle 1–3)

- ☐ Transitions
- ☐ Rhythm & Tempo
- ☐ Straightness
- ☐ Bend / Lateral Suppleness
- ☐ Engagement Behind
- ☐ Contact & Connection
- ☐ Adjustability / Stride Control
- ☐ Rideability / Focus
- ☐ Rider Position & Balance
- ☐ Jump Form / Gridwork

Notes:

Barn & Horse Management Notes

(Farrier, chiro, saddle fitter, health changes, shoeing, turnout, etc.)

Week of: _____

Weekly Training Plan

This Week's Goals

Horse Focus

_____

_____

_____

Rider Focus

_____

_____

_____

Conditioning & Schooling Schedule

(Examples: long and low day, cavaletti day, hill conditioning, lunge + stretch day)

Day	Plan / Exercise Focus	Notes
Mon	_____	_____
Tue	_____	_____
Wed	_____	_____
Thu	_____	_____
Fri	_____	_____
Sat	_____	_____
Sun	_____	_____

Primary Skill Focus This Week

(Check or circle 1–3)

- ☐ Transitions
- ☐ Rhythm & Tempo
- ☐ Straightness
- ☐ Bend / Lateral Suppleness
- ☐ Engagement Behind
- ☐ Contact & Connection
- ☐ Adjustability / Stride Control
- ☐ Rideability / Focus
- ☐ Rider Position & Balance
- ☐ Jump Form / Gridwork

Notes:

Barn & Horse Management Notes

(Farrier, chiro, saddle fitter, health changes, shoeing, turnout, etc.)

Week of: _____

Weekly Training Plan

This Week's Goals

Horse Focus

_____

_____

_____

Rider Focus

_____

_____

_____

Conditioning & Schooling Schedule

(Examples: long and low day, cavaletti day, hill conditioning, lunge + stretch day)

Day	Plan / Exercise Focus	Notes
Mon	_____	_____
Tue	_____	_____
Wed	_____	_____
Thu	_____	_____
Fri	_____	_____
Sat	_____	_____
Sun	_____	_____

Primary Skill Focus This Week

(Check or circle 1–3)

- ☐ Transitions
- ☐ Rhythm & Tempo
- ☐ Straightness
- ☐ Bend / Lateral Suppleness
- ☐ Engagement Behind
- ☐ Contact & Connection
- ☐ Adjustability / Stride Control
- ☐ Rideability / Focus
- ☐ Rider Position & Balance
- ☐ Jump Form / Gridwork

Notes:

Barn & Horse Management Notes

(Farrier, chiro, saddle fitter, health changes, shoeing, turnout, etc.)

Week of: _____

Weekly Training Plan

This Week's Goals

Horse Focus

_____

_____

_____

Rider Focus

_____

_____

_____

Conditioning & Schooling Schedule

(Examples: long and low day, cavaletti day, hill conditioning, lunge + stretch day)

Day	Plan / Exercise Focus	Notes
Mon	_____	_____
Tue	_____	_____
Wed	_____	_____
Thu	_____	_____
Fri	_____	_____
Sat	_____	_____
Sun	_____	_____

Primary Skill Focus This Week

(Check or circle 1–3)

- ☐ Transitions
- ☐ Rhythm & Tempo
- ☐ Straightness
- ☐ Bend / Lateral Suppleness
- ☐ Engagement Behind
- ☐ Contact & Connection
- ☐ Adjustability / Stride Control
- ☐ Rideability / Focus
- ☐ Rider Position & Balance
- ☐ Jump Form / Gridwork

Notes:

Barn & Horse Management Notes

(Farrier, chiro, saddle fitter, health changes, shoeing, turnout, etc.)

Week of: _____ *Weekly Training Plan*

This Week's Goals

Horse Focus

_____

_____

_____

Rider Focus

_____

_____

_____

Conditioning & Schooling Schedule

(Examples: long and low day, cavaletti day, hill conditioning, lunge + stretch day)

Day	Plan / Exercise Focus	Notes
Mon	_____	_____
Tue	_____	_____
Wed	_____	_____
Thu	_____	_____
Fri	_____	_____
Sat	_____	_____
Sun	_____	_____

Primary Skill Focus This Week

(Check or circle 1–3)

- ☐ Transitions
- ☐ Rhythm & Tempo
- ☐ Straightness
- ☐ Bend / Lateral Suppleness
- ☐ Engagement Behind
- ☐ Contact & Connection
- ☐ Adjustability / Stride Control
- ☐ Rideability / Focus
- ☐ Rider Position & Balance
- ☐ Jump Form / Gridwork

Notes:

Barn & Horse Management Notes

(Farrier, chiro, saddle fitter, health changes, shoeing, turnout, etc.)

Week of: _____ *Weekly Training Plan*

This Week's Goals

Horse Focus

_____

_____

_____

Rider Focus

_____

_____

_____

Conditioning & Schooling Schedule

(Examples: long and low day, cavaletti day, hill conditioning, lunge + stretch day)

Day	Plan / Exercise Focus	Notes
Mon	_____	_____
Tue	_____	_____
Wed	_____	_____
Thu	_____	_____
Fri	_____	_____
Sat	_____	_____
Sun	_____	_____

Primary Skill Focus This Week

(Check or circle 1–3)

- ☐ Transitions
- ☐ Rhythm & Tempo
- ☐ Straightness
- ☐ Bend / Lateral Suppleness
- ☐ Engagement Behind
- ☐ Contact & Connection
- ☐ Adjustability / Stride Control
- ☐ Rideability / Focus
- ☐ Rider Position & Balance
- ☐ Jump Form / Gridwork

Notes:

Barn & Horse Management Notes

(Farrier, chiro, saddle fitter, health changes, shoeing, turnout, etc.)

Week of: _____   *Weekly Training Plan*

This Week's Goals

Horse Focus

_____

_____

_____

Rider Focus

_____

_____

_____

Conditioning & Schooling Schedule

(Examples: long and low day, cavaletti day, hill conditioning, lunge + stretch day)

Day	Plan / Exercise Focus	Notes
Mon	_____	_____
Tue	_____	_____
Wed	_____	_____
Thu	_____	_____
Fri	_____	_____
Sat	_____	_____
Sun	_____	_____

Primary Skill Focus This Week

(Check or circle 1–3)

- ☐ Transitions
- ☐ Rhythm & Tempo
- ☐ Straightness
- ☐ Bend / Lateral Suppleness
- ☐ Engagement Behind
- ☐ Contact & Connection
- ☐ Adjustability / Stride Control
- ☐ Rideability / Focus
- ☐ Rider Position & Balance
- ☐ Jump Form / Gridwork

Notes:

Barn & Horse Management Notes

(Farrier, chiro, saddle fitter, health changes, shoeing, turnout, etc.)

Week of: _____ *Weekly Training Plan*

This Week's Goals

Horse Focus

_____

_____

_____

Rider Focus

_____

_____

_____

Conditioning & Schooling Schedule

(Examples: long and low day, cavaletti day, hill conditioning, lunge + stretch day)

Day	Plan / Exercise Focus	Notes
Mon	_____	_____
Tue	_____	_____
Wed	_____	_____
Thu	_____	_____
Fri	_____	_____
Sat	_____	_____
Sun	_____	_____

Primary Skill Focus This Week

(Check or circle 1–3)

- ☐ Transitions
- ☐ Rhythm & Tempo
- ☐ Straightness
- ☐ Bend / Lateral Suppleness
- ☐ Engagement Behind
- ☐ Contact & Connection
- ☐ Adjustability / Stride Control
- ☐ Rideability / Focus
- ☐ Rider Position & Balance
- ☐ Jump Form / Gridwork

Notes:

Barn & Horse Management Notes

(Farrier, chiro, saddle fitter, health changes, shoeing, turnout, etc.)

Week of: _____ *Weekly Training Plan*

This Week's Goals

Horse Focus

_____

_____

_____

Rider Focus

_____

_____

_____

Conditioning & Schooling Schedule

(Examples: long and low day, cavaletti day, hill conditioning, lunge + stretch day)

Day	Plan / Exercise Focus	Notes
Mon	_____	_____
Tue	_____	_____
Wed	_____	_____
Thu	_____	_____
Fri	_____	_____
Sat	_____	_____
Sun	_____	_____

Primary Skill Focus This Week

(Check or circle 1–3)

- ☐ Transitions
- ☐ Rhythm & Tempo
- ☐ Straightness
- ☐ Bend / Lateral Suppleness
- ☐ Engagement Behind
- ☐ Contact & Connection
- ☐ Adjustability / Stride Control
- ☐ Rideability / Focus
- ☐ Rider Position & Balance
- ☐ Jump Form / Gridwork

Notes:

Barn & Horse Management Notes

(Farrier, chiro, saddle fitter, health changes, shoeing, turnout, etc.)

Week of: _____   *Weekly Training Plan*

This Week's Goals

Horse Focus

_____

_____

_____

Rider Focus

_____

_____

_____

Conditioning & Schooling Schedule

(Examples: long and low day, cavaletti day, hill conditioning, lunge + stretch day)

Day	Plan / Exercise Focus	Notes
Mon	_____	_____
Tue	_____	_____
Wed	_____	_____
Thu	_____	_____
Fri	_____	_____
Sat	_____	_____
Sun	_____	_____

Primary Skill Focus This Week

(Check or circle 1–3)

- ☐ Transitions
- ☐ Rhythm & Tempo
- ☐ Straightness
- ☐ Bend / Lateral Suppleness
- ☐ Engagement Behind
- ☐ Contact & Connection
- ☐ Adjustability / Stride Control
- ☐ Rideability / Focus
- ☐ Rider Position & Balance
- ☐ Jump Form / Gridwork

Notes:

Barn & Horse Management Notes

(Farrier, chiro, saddle fitter, health changes, shoeing, turnout, etc.)

Weekly Training Plan

Week of: _____

This Week's Goals

Horse Focus

_____

_____

_____

Rider Focus

_____

_____

_____

Conditioning & Schooling Schedule

(Examples: long and low day, cavaletti day, hill conditioning, lunge + stretch day)

Day	Plan / Exercise Focus	Notes
Mon	_____	_____
Tue	_____	_____
Wed	_____	_____
Thu	_____	_____
Fri	_____	_____
Sat	_____	_____
Sun	_____	_____

Primary Skill Focus This Week

(Check or circle 1–3)

- ☐ Transitions
- ☐ Rhythm & Tempo
- ☐ Straightness
- ☐ Bend / Lateral Suppleness
- ☐ Engagement Behind
- ☐ Contact & Connection
- ☐ Adjustability / Stride Control
- ☐ Rideability / Focus
- ☐ Rider Position & Balance
- ☐ Jump Form / Gridwork

Notes:

Barn & Horse Management Notes

(Farrier, chiro, saddle fitter, health changes, shoeing, turnout, etc.)

Week of: _____ *Weekly Training Plan*

This Week's Goals

Horse Focus

_____

_____

_____

Rider Focus

_____

_____

_____

Conditioning & Schooling Schedule

(Examples: long and low day, cavaletti day, hill conditioning, lunge + stretch day)

Day	Plan / Exercise Focus	Notes
Mon	_____	_____
Tue	_____	_____
Wed	_____	_____
Thu	_____	_____
Fri	_____	_____
Sat	_____	_____
Sun	_____	_____

Primary Skill Focus This Week

(Check or circle 1–3)

- ☐ Transitions
- ☐ Rhythm & Tempo
- ☐ Straightness
- ☐ Bend / Lateral Suppleness
- ☐ Engagement Behind
- ☐ Contact & Connection
- ☐ Adjustability / Stride Control
- ☐ Rideability / Focus
- ☐ Rider Position & Balance
- ☐ Jump Form / Gridwork

Notes:

Barn & Horse Management Notes

(Farrier, chiro, saddle fitter, health changes, shoeing, turnout, etc.)

Week of: _____ *Weekly Training Plan*

This Week's Goals

Horse Focus

_____

_____

_____

Rider Focus

_____

_____

_____

Conditioning & Schooling Schedule

(Examples: long and low day, cavaletti day, hill conditioning, lunge + stretch day)

Day	Plan / Exercise Focus	Notes
Mon	_____	_____
Tue	_____	_____
Wed	_____	_____
Thu	_____	_____
Fri	_____	_____
Sat	_____	_____
Sun	_____	_____

Primary Skill Focus This Week

(Check or circle 1–3)

- ☐ Transitions
- ☐ Rhythm & Tempo
- ☐ Straightness
- ☐ Bend / Lateral Suppleness
- ☐ Engagement Behind
- ☐ Contact & Connection
- ☐ Adjustability / Stride Control
- ☐ Rideability / Focus
- ☐ Rider Position & Balance
- ☐ Jump Form / Gridwork

Notes:

Barn & Horse Management Notes

(Farrier, chiro, saddle fitter, health changes, shoeing, turnout, etc.)

Week of: _____

Weekly Training Plan

This Week's Goals

Horse Focus

_____

_____

_____

Rider Focus

_____

_____

_____

Conditioning & Schooling Schedule

(Examples: long and low day, cavaletti day, hill conditioning, lunge + stretch day)

Day	Plan / Exercise Focus	Notes
Mon	_____	_____
Tue	_____	_____
Wed	_____	_____
Thu	_____	_____
Fri	_____	_____
Sat	_____	_____
Sun	_____	_____

Primary Skill Focus This Week

(Check or circle 1–3)

- ☐ Transitions
- ☐ Rhythm & Tempo
- ☐ Straightness
- ☐ Bend / Lateral Suppleness
- ☐ Engagement Behind
- ☐ Contact & Connection
- ☐ Adjustability / Stride Control
- ☐ Rideability / Focus
- ☐ Rider Position & Balance
- ☐ Jump Form / Gridwork

Notes:

Barn & Horse Management Notes

(Farrier, chiro, saddle fitter, health changes, shoeing, turnout, etc.)

Week of: _____ *Weekly Training Plan*

This Week's Goals

Horse Focus

_____

_____

_____

Rider Focus

_____

_____

_____

Conditioning & Schooling Schedule

(Examples: long and low day, cavaletti day, hill conditioning, lunge + stretch day)

Day	Plan / Exercise Focus	Notes
Mon	_____	_____
Tue	_____	_____
Wed	_____	_____
Thu	_____	_____
Fri	_____	_____
Sat	_____	_____
Sun	_____	_____

Primary Skill Focus This Week

(Check or circle 1–3)

- ☐ Transitions
- ☐ Rhythm & Tempo
- ☐ Straightness
- ☐ Bend / Lateral Suppleness
- ☐ Engagement Behind
- ☐ Contact & Connection
- ☐ Adjustability / Stride Control
- ☐ Rideability / Focus
- ☐ Rider Position & Balance
- ☐ Jump Form / Gridwork

Notes:

Barn & Horse Management Notes

(Farrier, chiro, saddle fitter, health changes, shoeing, turnout, etc.)

Week of: _____ *Weekly Training Plan*

This Week's Goals

Horse Focus

_____

_____

_____

Rider Focus

_____

_____

_____

Conditioning & Schooling Schedule

(Examples: long and low day, cavaletti day, hill conditioning, lunge + stretch day)

Day	Plan / Exercise Focus	Notes
Mon	_____	_____
Tue	_____	_____
Wed	_____	_____
Thu	_____	_____
Fri	_____	_____
Sat	_____	_____
Sun	_____	_____

Primary Skill Focus This Week

(Check or circle 1–3)

- ☐ Transitions
- ☐ Rhythm & Tempo
- ☐ Straightness
- ☐ Bend / Lateral Suppleness
- ☐ Engagement Behind
- ☐ Contact & Connection
- ☐ Adjustability / Stride Control
- ☐ Rideability / Focus
- ☐ Rider Position & Balance
- ☐ Jump Form / Gridwork

Notes:

Barn & Horse Management Notes

(Farrier, chiro, saddle fitter, health changes, shoeing, turnout, etc.)

Week of: _____ *Weekly Training Plan*

This Week's Goals

Horse Focus

_____

_____

_____

Rider Focus

_____

_____

_____

Conditioning & Schooling Schedule

(Examples: long and low day, cavaletti day, hill conditioning, lunge + stretch day)

Day	Plan / Exercise Focus	Notes
Mon	_____	_____
Tue	_____	_____
Wed	_____	_____
Thu	_____	_____
Fri	_____	_____
Sat	_____	_____
Sun	_____	_____

Primary Skill Focus This Week

(Check or circle 1–3)

- ☐ Transitions
- ☐ Rhythm & Tempo
- ☐ Straightness
- ☐ Bend / Lateral Suppleness
- ☐ Engagement Behind
- ☐ Contact & Connection
- ☐ Adjustability / Stride Control
- ☐ Rideability / Focus
- ☐ Rider Position & Balance
- ☐ Jump Form / Gridwork

Notes:

Barn & Horse Management Notes

(Farrier, chiro, saddle fitter, health changes, shoeing, turnout, etc.)

Week of: _____ *Weekly Training Plan*

This Week's Goals

Horse Focus

_____

_____

_____

Rider Focus

_____

_____

_____

Conditioning & Schooling Schedule

(Examples: long and low day, cavaletti day, hill conditioning, lunge + stretch day)

Day	Plan / Exercise Focus	Notes
Mon	_____	_____
Tue	_____	_____
Wed	_____	_____
Thu	_____	_____
Fri	_____	_____
Sat	_____	_____
Sun	_____	_____

Primary Skill Focus This Week

(Check or circle 1–3)

- ☐ Transitions
- ☐ Rhythm & Tempo
- ☐ Straightness
- ☐ Bend / Lateral Suppleness
- ☐ Engagement Behind
- ☐ Contact & Connection
- ☐ Adjustability / Stride Control
- ☐ Rideability / Focus
- ☐ Rider Position & Balance
- ☐ Jump Form / Gridwork

Notes:

Barn & Horse Management Notes

(Farrier, chiro, saddle fitter, health changes, shoeing, turnout, etc.)

Week of: _____

Weekly Training Plan

This Week's Goals

Horse Focus

_____

_____

_____

Rider Focus

_____

_____

_____

Conditioning & Schooling Schedule

(Examples: long and low day, cavaletti day, hill conditioning, lunge + stretch day)

Day	Plan / Exercise Focus	Notes
Mon	_____	_____
Tue	_____	_____
Wed	_____	_____
Thu	_____	_____
Fri	_____	_____
Sat	_____	_____
Sun	_____	_____

Primary Skill Focus This Week

(Check or circle 1–3)

- ☐ Transitions
- ☐ Rhythm & Tempo
- ☐ Straightness
- ☐ Bend / Lateral Suppleness
- ☐ Engagement Behind
- ☐ Contact & Connection
- ☐ Adjustability / Stride Control
- ☐ Rideability / Focus
- ☐ Rider Position & Balance
- ☐ Jump Form / Gridwork

Notes:

Barn & Horse Management Notes

(Farrier, chiro, saddle fitter, health changes, shoeing, turnout, etc.)

Week of: _____ *Weekly Training Plan*

This Week's Goals

Horse Focus

_____

_____

_____

Rider Focus

_____

_____

_____

Conditioning & Schooling Schedule

(Examples: long and low day, cavaletti day, hill conditioning, lunge + stretch day)

Day	Plan / Exercise Focus	Notes
Mon	_____	_____
Tue	_____	_____
Wed	_____	_____
Thu	_____	_____
Fri	_____	_____
Sat	_____	_____
Sun	_____	_____

Primary Skill Focus This Week

(Check or circle 1–3)

- ☐ Transitions
- ☐ Rhythm & Tempo
- ☐ Straightness
- ☐ Bend / Lateral Suppleness
- ☐ Engagement Behind
- ☐ Contact & Connection
- ☐ Adjustability / Stride Control
- ☐ Rideability / Focus
- ☐ Rider Position & Balance
- ☐ Jump Form / Gridwork

Notes:

Barn & Horse Management Notes

(Farrier, chiro, saddle fitter, health changes, shoeing, turnout, etc.)

Week of: _____ *Weekly Training Plan*

This Week's Goals

Horse Focus

_____

_____

_____

Rider Focus

_____

_____

_____

Conditioning & Schooling Schedule

(Examples: long and low day, cavaletti day, hill conditioning, lunge + stretch day)

Day	Plan / Exercise Focus	Notes
Mon	_____	_____
Tue	_____	_____
Wed	_____	_____
Thu	_____	_____
Fri	_____	_____
Sat	_____	_____
Sun	_____	_____

Primary Skill Focus This Week

(Check or circle 1–3)

- ☐ Transitions
- ☐ Rhythm & Tempo
- ☐ Straightness
- ☐ Bend / Lateral Suppleness
- ☐ Engagement Behind
- ☐ Contact & Connection
- ☐ Adjustability / Stride Control
- ☐ Rideability / Focus
- ☐ Rider Position & Balance
- ☐ Jump Form / Gridwork

Notes:

Barn & Horse Management Notes

(Farrier, chiro, saddle fitter, health changes, shoeing, turnout, etc.)

Week of: _____ *Weekly Training Plan*

This Week's Goals

Horse Focus

_____

_____

_____

Rider Focus

_____

_____

_____

Conditioning & Schooling Schedule

(Examples: long and low day, cavaletti day, hill conditioning, lunge + stretch day)

Day	Plan / Exercise Focus	Notes
Mon	_____	_____
Tue	_____	_____
Wed	_____	_____
Thu	_____	_____
Fri	_____	_____
Sat	_____	_____
Sun	_____	_____

Primary Skill Focus This Week

(Check or circle 1–3)

- ☐ Transitions
- ☐ Rhythm & Tempo
- ☐ Straightness
- ☐ Bend / Lateral Suppleness
- ☐ Engagement Behind
- ☐ Contact & Connection
- ☐ Adjustability / Stride Control
- ☐ Rideability / Focus
- ☐ Rider Position & Balance
- ☐ Jump Form / Gridwork

Notes:

Barn & Horse Management Notes

(Farrier, chiro, saddle fitter, health changes, shoeing, turnout, etc.)

Week of: _____ *Weekly Training Plan*

This Week's Goals

Horse Focus

_____

_____

_____

Rider Focus

_____

_____

_____

Conditioning & Schooling Schedule

(Examples: long and low day, cavaletti day, hill conditioning, lunge + stretch day)

Day	Plan / Exercise Focus	Notes
Mon	_____	_____
Tue	_____	_____
Wed	_____	_____
Thu	_____	_____
Fri	_____	_____
Sat	_____	_____
Sun	_____	_____

Primary Skill Focus This Week

(Check or circle 1–3)

- ☐ Transitions
- ☐ Rhythm & Tempo
- ☐ Straightness
- ☐ Bend / Lateral Suppleness
- ☐ Engagement Behind
- ☐ Contact & Connection
- ☐ Adjustability / Stride Control
- ☐ Rideability / Focus
- ☐ Rider Position & Balance
- ☐ Jump Form / Gridwork

Notes:

Barn & Horse Management Notes

(Farrier, chiro, saddle fitter, health changes, shoeing, turnout, etc.)

Week of: _____ *Weekly Training Plan*

This Week's Goals

Horse Focus

_____

_____

_____

Rider Focus

_____

_____

_____

Conditioning & Schooling Schedule

(Examples: long and low day, cavaletti day, hill conditioning, lunge + stretch day)

Day	Plan / Exercise Focus	Notes
Mon	_____	_____
Tue	_____	_____
Wed	_____	_____
Thu	_____	_____
Fri	_____	_____
Sat	_____	_____
Sun	_____	_____

Primary Skill Focus This Week

(Check or circle 1–3)

- ☐ Transitions
- ☐ Rhythm & Tempo
- ☐ Straightness
- ☐ Bend / Lateral Suppleness
- ☐ Engagement Behind
- ☐ Contact & Connection
- ☐ Adjustability / Stride Control
- ☐ Rideability / Focus
- ☐ Rider Position & Balance
- ☐ Jump Form / Gridwork

Notes:

Barn & Horse Management Notes

(Farrier, chiro, saddle fitter, health changes, shoeing, turnout, etc.)

Weekly Training Plan

Week of: _____

This Week's Goals

Horse Focus

_____

_____

_____

Rider Focus

_____

_____

_____

Conditioning & Schooling Schedule

(Examples: long and low day, cavaletti day, hill conditioning, lunge + stretch day)

Day	Plan / Exercise Focus	Notes
Mon	_____	_____
Tue	_____	_____
Wed	_____	_____
Thu	_____	_____
Fri	_____	_____
Sat	_____	_____
Sun	_____	_____

Primary Skill Focus This Week

(Check or circle 1–3)

- ☐ Transitions
- ☐ Rhythm & Tempo
- ☐ Straightness
- ☐ Bend / Lateral Suppleness
- ☐ Engagement Behind
- ☐ Contact & Connection
- ☐ Adjustability / Stride Control
- ☐ Rideability / Focus
- ☐ Rider Position & Balance
- ☐ Jump Form / Gridwork

Notes:

Barn & Horse Management Notes

(Farrier, chiro, saddle fitter, health changes, shoeing, turnout, etc.)

Week of: _____   *Weekly Training Plan*

This Week's Goals

Horse Focus

_____

_____

_____

Rider Focus

_____

_____

_____

Conditioning & Schooling Schedule

(Examples: long and low day, cavaletti day, hill conditioning, lunge + stretch day)

Day	Plan / Exercise Focus	Notes
Mon	_____	_____
Tue	_____	_____
Wed	_____	_____
Thu	_____	_____
Fri	_____	_____
Sat	_____	_____
Sun	_____	_____

Primary Skill Focus This Week

(Check or circle 1–3)

- ☐ Transitions
- ☐ Rhythm & Tempo
- ☐ Straightness
- ☐ Bend / Lateral Suppleness
- ☐ Engagement Behind
- ☐ Contact & Connection
- ☐ Adjustability / Stride Control
- ☐ Rideability / Focus
- ☐ Rider Position & Balance
- ☐ Jump Form / Gridwork

Notes:

Barn & Horse Management Notes

(Farrier, chiro, saddle fitter, health changes, shoeing, turnout, etc.)

Week of: _____   *Weekly Training Plan*

This Week's Goals

Horse Focus

_____

_____

_____

Rider Focus

_____

_____

_____

Conditioning & Schooling Schedule

(Examples: long and low day, cavaletti day, hill conditioning, lunge + stretch day)

Day	Plan / Exercise Focus	Notes
Mon	_____	_____
Tue	_____	_____
Wed	_____	_____
Thu	_____	_____
Fri	_____	_____
Sat	_____	_____
Sun	_____	_____

Primary Skill Focus This Week

(Check or circle 1–3)

- ☐ Transitions
- ☐ Rhythm & Tempo
- ☐ Straightness
- ☐ Bend / Lateral Suppleness
- ☐ Engagement Behind
- ☐ Contact & Connection
- ☐ Adjustability / Stride Control
- ☐ Rideability / Focus
- ☐ Rider Position & Balance
- ☐ Jump Form / Gridwork

Notes:

Barn & Horse Management Notes

(Farrier, chiro, saddle fitter, health changes, shoeing, turnout, etc.)

Week of: _____   # Weekly Training Plan

This Week's Goals

Horse Focus

_____

_____

_____

Rider Focus

_____

_____

_____

Conditioning & Schooling Schedule

(Examples: long and low day, cavaletti day, hill conditioning, lunge + stretch day)

Day	Plan / Exercise Focus	Notes
Mon	_____	_____
Tue	_____	_____
Wed	_____	_____
Thu	_____	_____
Fri	_____	_____
Sat	_____	_____

Primary Skill Focus This Week

(Check or circle 1–3)

- ☐ Transitions
- ☐ Rhythm & Tempo
- ☐ Straightness
- ☐ Bend / Lateral Suppleness
- ☐ Engagement Behind
- ☐ Contact & Connection
- ☐ Adjustability / Stride Control
- ☐ Rideability / Focus
- ☐ Rider Position & Balance
- ☐ Jump Form / Gridwork

Notes:

_____

_____

Barn & Horse Management Notes

(Farrier, chiro, saddle fitter, health changes, shoeing, turnout, etc.)

Daily Schooling Session Log

Daily Schooling Session Log

Date: _____ Horse: _____   Date: _____ Horse: _____

Warm-Up

What did you do? How did the horse feel?

Warm-Up

What did you do? How did the horse feel?

Focused Exercises

Flatwork Goals

_____

_____

_____

Focused Exercises

Flatwork Goals

_____

_____

_____

Breakthroughs / Things That Went Well

Breakthroughs / Things That Went Well

Resistance / Challenges

Resistance / Challenges

Cool-Down Notes

Cool-Down Notes

Homework / Drills for Next Time

Homework / Drills for Next Time

Daily Schooling Session Log

Date: _____   Horse: _____   Date: _____   Horse: _____

Warm-Up

What did you do? How did the horse feel?

Warm-Up

What did you do? How did the horse feel?

Focused Exercises

Flatwork Goals

_____

_____

_____

Focused Exercises

Flatwork Goals

_____

_____

_____

Breakthroughs / Things That Went Well

Breakthroughs / Things That Went Well

Resistance / Challenges

Resistance / Challenges

Cool-Down Notes

Cool-Down Notes

Homework / Drills for Next Time

Homework / Drills for Next Time

Daily Schooling Session Log

Date: _____   Horse: _____   Date: _____   Horse: _____

Warm-Up

What did you do? How did the horse feel?

Warm-Up

What did you do? How did the horse feel?

Focused Exercises

Flatwork Goals

_____

_____

_____

Focused Exercises

Flatwork Goals

_____

_____

_____

Breakthroughs / Things That Went Well

Breakthroughs / Things That Went Well

Resistance / Challenges

Resistance / Challenges

Cool-Down Notes

Cool-Down Notes

Homework / Drills for Next Time

Homework / Drills for Next Time

Daily Schooling Session Log

Date: _____   Horse: _____   Date: _____   Horse: _____

Warm-Up

What did you do? How did the horse feel?

Warm-Up

What did you do? How did the horse feel?

Focused Exercises

Flatwork Goals

_____

_____

_____

Focused Exercises

Flatwork Goals

_____

_____

_____

Breakthroughs / Things That Went Well

Breakthroughs / Things That Went Well

Resistance / Challenges

Resistance / Challenges

Cool-Down Notes

Cool-Down Notes

Homework / Drills for Next Time

Homework / Drills for Next Time

Daily Schooling Session Log

Date: _____   Horse: _____   Date: _____   Horse: _____

Warm-Up

What did you do? How did the horse feel?

Warm-Up

What did you do? How did the horse feel?

Focused Exercises

Flatwork Goals

_____

_____

_____

Focused Exercises

Flatwork Goals

_____

_____

_____

Breakthroughs / Things That Went Well

Breakthroughs / Things That Went Well

Resistance / Challenges

Resistance / Challenges

Cool-Down Notes

Cool-Down Notes

Homework / Drills for Next Time

Homework / Drills for Next Time

Daily Schooling Session Log

Date: _____   Horse: _____   Date: _____   Horse: _____

Warm-Up

What did you do? How did the horse feel?

Warm-Up

What did you do? How did the horse feel?

Focused Exercises

Flatwork Goals

_____

_____

_____

Focused Exercises

Flatwork Goals

_____

_____

_____

Breakthroughs / Things That Went Well

Breakthroughs / Things That Went Well

Resistance / Challenges

Resistance / Challenges

Cool-Down Notes

Cool-Down Notes

Homework / Drills for Next Time

Homework / Drills for Next Time

Daily Schooling Session Log

Date: _____   Horse: _____   Date: _____   Horse: _____

Warm-Up

What did you do? How did the horse feel?

Warm-Up

What did you do? How did the horse feel?

Focused Exercises

Flatwork Goals

_____

_____

_____

Focused Exercises

Flatwork Goals

_____

_____

_____

Breakthroughs / Things That Went Well

Breakthroughs / Things That Went Well

Resistance / Challenges

Resistance / Challenges

Cool-Down Notes

Cool-Down Notes

Homework / Drills for Next Time

Homework / Drills for Next Time

Daily Schooling Session Log

Date: _____   Horse: _____   Date: _____   Horse: _____

Warm-Up

What did you do? How did the horse feel?

Warm-Up

What did you do? How did the horse feel?

Focused Exercises

Flatwork Goals

_____

_____

_____

Focused Exercises

Flatwork Goals

_____

_____

_____

Breakthroughs / Things That Went Well

Breakthroughs / Things That Went Well

Resistance / Challenges

Resistance / Challenges

Cool-Down Notes

Cool-Down Notes

Homework / Drills for Next Time

Homework / Drills for Next Time

Daily Schooling Session Log

Date: _____ Horse: _____   Date: _____ Horse: _____

Warm-Up

What did you do? How did the horse feel?

Warm-Up

What did you do? How did the horse feel?

Focused Exercises

Flatwork Goals

_____

_____

_____

Focused Exercises

Flatwork Goals

_____

_____

_____

Breakthroughs / Things That Went Well

Breakthroughs / Things That Went Well

Resistance / Challenges

Resistance / Challenges

Cool-Down Notes

Cool-Down Notes

Homework / Drills for Next Time

Homework / Drills for Next Time

Daily Schooling Session Log

Date: _____ Horse: _____   Date: _____ Horse: _____

Warm-Up

What did you do? How did the horse feel?

Warm-Up

What did you do? How did the horse feel?

Focused Exercises

Flatwork Goals

_____

_____

_____

Focused Exercises

Flatwork Goals

_____

_____

_____

Breakthroughs / Things That Went Well

Breakthroughs / Things That Went Well

Resistance / Challenges

Resistance / Challenges

Cool-Down Notes

Cool-Down Notes

Homework / Drills for Next Time

Homework / Drills for Next Time

Daily Schooling Session Log

Date: _____ Horse: _____   Date: _____ Horse: _____

Warm-Up

What did you do? How did the horse feel?

Warm-Up

What did you do? How did the horse feel?

Focused Exercises

Flatwork Goals

_____

_____

_____

Focused Exercises

Flatwork Goals

_____

_____

_____

Breakthroughs / Things That Went Well

Breakthroughs / Things That Went Well

Resistance / Challenges

Resistance / Challenges

Cool-Down Notes

Cool-Down Notes

Homework / Drills for Next Time

Homework / Drills for Next Time

Daily Schooling Session Log

Date: _____ Horse: _____   Date: _____ Horse: _____

Warm-Up

What did you do? How did the horse feel?

Warm-Up

What did you do? How did the horse feel?

Focused Exercises

Flatwork Goals

_____

_____

_____

Focused Exercises

Flatwork Goals

_____

_____

_____

Breakthroughs / Things That Went Well

Breakthroughs / Things That Went Well

Resistance / Challenges

Resistance / Challenges

Cool-Down Notes

Cool-Down Notes

Homework / Drills for Next Time

Homework / Drills for Next Time

Daily Schooling Session Log

Date: _____   Horse: _____   Date: _____   Horse: _____

Warm-Up

What did you do? How did the horse feel?

Warm-Up

What did you do? How did the horse feel?

Focused Exercises

Flatwork Goals

_____

_____

_____

Focused Exercises

Flatwork Goals

_____

_____

_____

Breakthroughs / Things That Went Well

Breakthroughs / Things That Went Well

Resistance / Challenges

Resistance / Challenges

Cool-Down Notes

Cool-Down Notes

Homework / Drills for Next Time

Homework / Drills for Next Time

Daily Schooling Session Log

Date: _____   Horse: _____   Date: _____   Horse: _____

Warm-Up

What did you do? How did the horse feel?

Warm-Up

What did you do? How did the horse feel?

Focused Exercises

Flatwork Goals

_____

_____

_____

Focused Exercises

Flatwork Goals

_____

_____

_____

Breakthroughs / Things That Went Well

Breakthroughs / Things That Went Well

Resistance / Challenges

Resistance / Challenges

Cool-Down Notes

Cool-Down Notes

Homework / Drills for Next Time

Homework / Drills for Next Time

Daily Schooling Session Log

Date: _____ Horse: _____   Date: _____ Horse: _____

Warm-Up

What did you do? How did the horse feel?

Warm-Up

What did you do? How did the horse feel?

Focused Exercises

Flatwork Goals

_____

_____

_____

Focused Exercises

Flatwork Goals

_____

_____

_____

Breakthroughs / Things That Went Well

Breakthroughs / Things That Went Well

Resistance / Challenges

Resistance / Challenges

Cool-Down Notes

Cool-Down Notes

Homework / Drills for Next Time

Homework / Drills for Next Time

Daily Schooling Session Log

Date: _____   Horse: _____   Date: _____   Horse: _____

Warm-Up

What did you do? How did the horse feel?

Warm-Up

What did you do? How did the horse feel?

Focused Exercises

Flatwork Goals

_____

_____

_____

Focused Exercises

Flatwork Goals

_____

_____

_____

Breakthroughs / Things That Went Well

Breakthroughs / Things That Went Well

Resistance / Challenges

Resistance / Challenges

Cool-Down Notes

Cool-Down Notes

Homework / Drills for Next Time

Homework / Drills for Next Time

Daily Schooling Session Log

Date: _____   Horse: _____   Date: _____   Horse: _____

Warm-Up

What did you do? How did the horse feel?

Warm-Up

What did you do? How did the horse feel?

Focused Exercises

Flatwork Goals

_____

_____

_____

Focused Exercises

Flatwork Goals

_____

_____

_____

Breakthroughs / Things That Went Well

Breakthroughs / Things That Went Well

Resistance / Challenges

Resistance / Challenges

Cool-Down Notes

Cool-Down Notes

Homework / Drills for Next Time

Homework / Drills for Next Time

Daily Schooling Session Log

Date: _____ Horse: _____ Date: _____ Horse: _____

Warm-Up

What did you do? How did the horse feel?

Warm-Up

What did you do? How did the horse feel?

Focused Exercises

Flatwork Goals

_____

_____

_____

Focused Exercises

Flatwork Goals

_____

_____

_____

Breakthroughs / Things That Went Well

Breakthroughs / Things That Went Well

Resistance / Challenges

Resistance / Challenges

Cool-Down Notes

Cool-Down Notes

Homework / Drills for Next Time

Homework / Drills for Next Time

Daily Schooling Session Log

Date: _____ Horse: _____   Date: _____ Horse: _____

Warm-Up
What did you do? How did the horse feel?

Warm-Up
What did you do? How did the horse feel?

Focused Exercises
Flatwork Goals

_____

_____

_____

Focused Exercises
Flatwork Goals

_____

_____

_____

Breakthroughs / Things That Went Well

Breakthroughs / Things That Went Well

Resistance / Challenges

Resistance / Challenges

Cool-Down Notes

Cool-Down Notes

Homework / Drills for Next Time

Homework / Drills for Next Time

Daily Schooling Session Log

Date: _____   Horse: _____   Date: _____   Horse: _____

Warm-Up

What did you do? How did the horse feel?

Warm-Up

What did you do? How did the horse feel?

Focused Exercises

Flatwork Goals

_____

_____

_____

Focused Exercises

Flatwork Goals

_____

_____

_____

Breakthroughs / Things That Went Well

Breakthroughs / Things That Went Well

Resistance / Challenges

Resistance / Challenges

Cool-Down Notes

Cool-Down Notes

Homework / Drills for Next Time

Homework / Drills for Next Time

Daily Schooling Session Log

Date: _____ Horse: _____   Date: _____ Horse: _____

Warm-Up

What did you do? How did the horse feel?

Warm-Up

What did you do? How did the horse feel?

Focused Exercises

Flatwork Goals

_____

_____

_____

Focused Exercises

Flatwork Goals

_____

_____

_____

Breakthroughs / Things That Went Well

Breakthroughs / Things That Went Well

Resistance / Challenges

Resistance / Challenges

Cool-Down Notes

Cool-Down Notes

Homework / Drills for Next Time

Homework / Drills for Next Time

Daily Schooling Session Log

Date: _____ Horse: _____   Date: _____ Horse: _____

Warm-Up

What did you do? How did the horse feel?

Warm-Up

What did you do? How did the horse feel?

Focused Exercises

Flatwork Goals

_____

_____

_____

Focused Exercises

Flatwork Goals

_____

_____

_____

Breakthroughs / Things That Went Well

Breakthroughs / Things That Went Well

Resistance / Challenges

Resistance / Challenges

Cool-Down Notes

Cool-Down Notes

Homework / Drills for Next Time

Homework / Drills for Next Time

Daily Schooling Session Log

Date: _____ Horse: _____   Date: _____ Horse: _____

Warm-Up

What did you do? How did the horse feel?

Warm-Up

What did you do? How did the horse feel?

Focused Exercises

Flatwork Goals

_____

_____

_____

Focused Exercises

Flatwork Goals

_____

_____

_____

Breakthroughs / Things That Went Well

Breakthroughs / Things That Went Well

Resistance / Challenges

Resistance / Challenges

Cool-Down Notes

Cool-Down Notes

Homework / Drills for Next Time

Homework / Drills for Next Time

Daily Schooling Session Log

Date: _____ Horse: _____   Date: _____ Horse: _____

Warm-Up

What did you do? How did the horse feel?

Warm-Up

What did you do? How did the horse feel?

Focused Exercises

Flatwork Goals

_____

_____

_____

Focused Exercises

Flatwork Goals

_____

_____

_____

Breakthroughs / Things That Went Well

Breakthroughs / Things That Went Well

Resistance / Challenges

Resistance / Challenges

Cool-Down Notes

Cool-Down Notes

Homework / Drills for Next Time

Homework / Drills for Next Time

Daily Schooling Session Log

Date: _____   Horse: _____   Date: _____   Horse: _____

Warm-Up

What did you do? How did the horse feel?

Warm-Up

What did you do? How did the horse feel?

Focused Exercises

Flatwork Goals

_____

_____

_____

Focused Exercises

Flatwork Goals

_____

_____

_____

Breakthroughs / Things That Went Well

Breakthroughs / Things That Went Well

Resistance / Challenges

Resistance / Challenges

Cool-Down Notes

Cool-Down Notes

Homework / Drills for Next Time

Homework / Drills for Next Time

Daily Schooling Session Log

Date: _____   Horse: _____   Date: _____   Horse: _____

Warm-Up

What did you do? How did the horse feel?

Warm-Up

What did you do? How did the horse feel?

Focused Exercises

Flatwork Goals

_____

_____

_____

Focused Exercises

Flatwork Goals

_____

_____

_____

Breakthroughs / Things That Went Well

Breakthroughs / Things That Went Well

Resistance / Challenges

Resistance / Challenges

Cool-Down Notes

Cool-Down Notes

Homework / Drills for Next Time

Homework / Drills for Next Time

Daily Schooling Session Log

Date: _____   Horse: _____   Date: _____   Horse: _____

Warm-Up
What did you do? How did the horse feel?

Warm-Up
What did you do? How did the horse feel?

Focused Exercises
Flatwork Goals

_____

_____

_____

Focused Exercises
Flatwork Goals

_____

_____

_____

Breakthroughs / Things That Went Well

Breakthroughs / Things That Went Well

Resistance / Challenges

Resistance / Challenges

Cool-Down Notes

Cool-Down Notes

Homework / Drills for Next Time

Homework / Drills for Next Time

Daily Schooling Session Log

Date: _____   Horse: _____   Date: _____   Horse: _____

Warm-Up

What did you do? How did the horse feel?

Warm-Up

What did you do? How did the horse feel?

Focused Exercises

Flatwork Goals

_____

_____

_____

Focused Exercises

Flatwork Goals

_____

_____

_____

Breakthroughs / Things That Went Well

Breakthroughs / Things That Went Well

Resistance / Challenges

Resistance / Challenges

Cool-Down Notes

Cool-Down Notes

Homework / Drills for Next Time

Homework / Drills for Next Time

Daily Schooling Session Log

Date: _____   Horse: _____   Date: _____   Horse: _____

Warm-Up

What did you do? How did the horse feel?

Warm-Up

What did you do? How did the horse feel?

Focused Exercises

Flatwork Goals

_____

_____

_____

Focused Exercises

Flatwork Goals

_____

_____

_____

Breakthroughs / Things That Went Well

Breakthroughs / Things That Went Well

Resistance / Challenges

Resistance / Challenges

Cool-Down Notes

Cool-Down Notes

Homework / Drills for Next Time

Homework / Drills for Next Time

Daily Schooling Session Log

Date: _____   Horse: _____   Date: _____   Horse: _____

Warm-Up

What did you do? How did the horse feel?

Warm-Up

What did you do? How did the horse feel?

Focused Exercises

Flatwork Goals

_____

_____

_____

Focused Exercises

Flatwork Goals

_____

_____

_____

Breakthroughs / Things That Went Well

Breakthroughs / Things That Went Well

Resistance / Challenges

Resistance / Challenges

Cool-Down Notes

Cool-Down Notes

Homework / Drills for Next Time

Homework / Drills for Next Time

Daily Schooling Session Log

Date: _____   Horse: _____   Date: _____   Horse: _____

Warm-Up
What did you do? How did the horse feel?

Warm-Up
What did you do? How did the horse feel?

Focused Exercises

Flatwork Goals

_____

_____

_____

Focused Exercises

Flatwork Goals

_____

_____

_____

Breakthroughs / Things That Went Well

Breakthroughs / Things That Went Well

Resistance / Challenges

Resistance / Challenges

Cool-Down Notes

Cool-Down Notes

Homework / Drills for Next Time

Homework / Drills for Next Time

Daily Schooling Session Log

Date: _____ Horse: _____   Date: _____ Horse: _____

Warm-Up
What did you do? How did the horse feel?

Warm-Up
What did you do? How did the horse feel?

Focused Exercises
Flatwork Goals

_____

_____

_____

Focused Exercises
Flatwork Goals

_____

_____

_____

Breakthroughs / Things That Went Well

Breakthroughs / Things That Went Well

Resistance / Challenges

Resistance / Challenges

Cool-Down Notes

Cool-Down Notes

Homework / Drills for Next Time

Homework / Drills for Next Time

Daily Schooling Session Log

Date: _____ Horse: _____   Date: _____ Horse: _____

Warm-Up

What did you do? How did the horse feel?

Warm-Up

What did you do? How did the horse feel?

Focused Exercises

Flatwork Goals

_____

_____

_____

Focused Exercises

Flatwork Goals

_____

_____

_____

Breakthroughs / Things That Went Well

Breakthroughs / Things That Went Well

Resistance / Challenges

Resistance / Challenges

Cool-Down Notes

Cool-Down Notes

Homework / Drills for Next Time

Homework / Drills for Next Time

Daily Schooling Session Log

Date: _____ Horse: _____   Date: _____ Horse: _____

Warm-Up

What did you do? How did the horse feel?

Warm-Up

What did you do? How did the horse feel?

Focused Exercises

Flatwork Goals

_____

_____

_____

Focused Exercises

Flatwork Goals

_____

_____

_____

Breakthroughs / Things That Went Well

Breakthroughs / Things That Went Well

Resistance / Challenges

Resistance / Challenges

Cool-Down Notes

Cool-Down Notes

Homework / Drills for Next Time

Homework / Drills for Next Time

Daily Schooling Session Log

Date: _____   Horse: _____   Date: _____   Horse: _____

Warm-Up

What did you do? How did the horse feel?

Warm-Up

What did you do? How did the horse feel?

Focused Exercises

Flatwork Goals

_____

_____

_____

Focused Exercises

Flatwork Goals

_____

_____

_____

Breakthroughs / Things That Went Well

Breakthroughs / Things That Went Well

Resistance / Challenges

Resistance / Challenges

Cool-Down Notes

Cool-Down Notes

Homework / Drills for Next Time

Homework / Drills for Next Time

Daily Schooling Session Log

Date: _____   Horse: _____   Date: _____   Horse: _____

Warm-Up

What did you do? How did the horse feel?

Warm-Up

What did you do? How did the horse feel?

Focused Exercises

Flatwork Goals

_____

_____

_____

Focused Exercises

Flatwork Goals

_____

_____

_____

Breakthroughs / Things That Went Well

Breakthroughs / Things That Went Well

Resistance / Challenges

Resistance / Challenges

Cool-Down Notes

Cool-Down Notes

Homework / Drills for Next Time

Homework / Drills for Next Time

Daily Schooling Session Log

Date: _____ Horse: _____   Date: _____ Horse: _____

Warm-Up

What did you do? How did the horse feel?

Warm-Up

What did you do? How did the horse feel?

Focused Exercises

Flatwork Goals

_____

_____

_____

Focused Exercises

Flatwork Goals

_____

_____

_____

Breakthroughs / Things That Went Well

Breakthroughs / Things That Went Well

Resistance / Challenges

Resistance / Challenges

Cool-Down Notes

Cool-Down Notes

Homework / Drills for Next Time

Homework / Drills for Next Time

Daily Schooling Session Log

Date: _____ Horse: _____   Date: _____ Horse: _____

Warm-Up

What did you do? How did the horse feel?

Warm-Up

What did you do? How did the horse feel?

Focused Exercises

Flatwork Goals

_____

_____

_____

Focused Exercises

Flatwork Goals

_____

_____

_____

Breakthroughs / Things That Went Well

Breakthroughs / Things That Went Well

Resistance / Challenges

Resistance / Challenges

Cool-Down Notes

Cool-Down Notes

Homework / Drills for Next Time

Homework / Drills for Next Time

Daily Schooling Session Log

Date: _____   Horse: _____   Date: _____   Horse: _____

Warm-Up

What did you do? How did the horse feel?

Warm-Up

What did you do? How did the horse feel?

Focused Exercises

Flatwork Goals

_____

_____

_____

Focused Exercises

Flatwork Goals

_____

_____

_____

Breakthroughs / Things That Went Well

Breakthroughs / Things That Went Well

Resistance / Challenges

Resistance / Challenges

Cool-Down Notes

Cool-Down Notes

Homework / Drills for Next Time

Homework / Drills for Next Time

Daily Schooling Session Log

Date: _____   Horse: _____   Date: _____   Horse: _____

Warm-Up

What did you do? How did the horse feel?

Warm-Up

What did you do? How did the horse feel?

Focused Exercises

Flatwork Goals

_____

_____

_____

Focused Exercises

Flatwork Goals

_____

_____

_____

Breakthroughs / Things That Went Well

Breakthroughs / Things That Went Well

Resistance / Challenges

Resistance / Challenges

Cool-Down Notes

Cool-Down Notes

Homework / Drills for Next Time

Homework / Drills for Next Time

Daily Schooling Session Log

Date: _____   Horse: _____   Date: _____   Horse: _____

Warm-Up

What did you do? How did the horse feel?

Warm-Up

What did you do? How did the horse feel?

Focused Exercises

Flatwork Goals

_____

_____

_____

Focused Exercises

Flatwork Goals

_____

_____

_____

Breakthroughs / Things That Went Well

Breakthroughs / Things That Went Well

Resistance / Challenges

Resistance / Challenges

Cool-Down Notes

Cool-Down Notes

Homework / Drills for Next Time

Homework / Drills for Next Time

Daily Schooling Session Log

Date: _____   Horse: _____   Date: _____   Horse: _____

Warm-Up

What did you do? How did the horse feel?

Warm-Up

What did you do? How did the horse feel?

Focused Exercises

Flatwork Goals

_____

_____

_____

Focused Exercises

Flatwork Goals

_____

_____

_____

Breakthroughs / Things That Went Well

Breakthroughs / Things That Went Well

Resistance / Challenges

Resistance / Challenges

Cool-Down Notes

Cool-Down Notes

Homework / Drills for Next Time

Homework / Drills for Next Time

Daily Schooling Session Log

Date: _____ Horse: _____   Date: _____ Horse: _____

Warm-Up

What did you do? How did the horse feel?

Warm-Up

What did you do? How did the horse feel?

Focused Exercises

Flatwork Goals

_____

_____

_____

Focused Exercises

Flatwork Goals

_____

_____

_____

Breakthroughs / Things That Went Well

Breakthroughs / Things That Went Well

Resistance / Challenges

Resistance / Challenges

Cool-Down Notes

Cool-Down Notes

Homework / Drills for Next Time

Homework / Drills for Next Time

Daily Schooling Session Log

Date: _____ Horse: _____   Date: _____ Horse: _____

Warm-Up

What did you do? How did the horse feel?

Warm-Up

What did you do? How did the horse feel?

Focused Exercises

Flatwork Goals

_____

_____

_____

Focused Exercises

Flatwork Goals

_____

_____

_____

Breakthroughs / Things That Went Well

Breakthroughs / Things That Went Well

Resistance / Challenges

Resistance / Challenges

Cool-Down Notes

Cool-Down Notes

Homework / Drills for Next Time

Homework / Drills for Next Time

Daily Schooling Session Log

Date: _____ Horse: _____   Date: _____ Horse: _____

Warm-Up

What did you do? How did the horse feel?

Warm-Up

What did you do? How did the horse feel?

Focused Exercises

Flatwork Goals

_____

_____

_____

Focused Exercises

Flatwork Goals

_____

_____

_____

Breakthroughs / Things That Went Well

Breakthroughs / Things That Went Well

Resistance / Challenges

Resistance / Challenges

Cool-Down Notes

Cool-Down Notes

Homework / Drills for Next Time

Homework / Drills for Next Time

Daily Schooling Session Log

Date: _____   Horse: _____   Date: _____   Horse: _____

Warm-Up

What did you do? How did the horse feel?

Focused Exercises

Flatwork Goals

_____

_____

_____

Breakthroughs / Things That Went Well

Resistance / Challenges

Cool-Down Notes

Homework / Drills for Next Time

Warm-Up

What did you do? How did the horse feel?

Focused Exercises

Flatwork Goals

_____

_____

_____

Breakthroughs / Things That Went Well

Resistance / Challenges

Cool-Down Notes

Homework / Drills for Next Time

Daily Schooling Session Log

Date: _____   Horse: _____   Date: _____   Horse: _____

Warm-Up

What did you do? How did the horse feel?

Warm-Up

What did you do? How did the horse feel?

Focused Exercises

Flatwork Goals

_____

_____

_____

Focused Exercises

Flatwork Goals

_____

_____

_____

Breakthroughs / Things That Went Well

Breakthroughs / Things That Went Well

Resistance / Challenges

Resistance / Challenges

Cool-Down Notes

Cool-Down Notes

Homework / Drills for Next Time

Homework / Drills for Next Time

Daily Schooling Session Log

Date: _____   Horse: _____   Date: _____   Horse: _____

Warm-Up

What did you do? How did the horse feel?

Focused Exercises

Flatwork Goals

_____

_____

_____

Breakthroughs / Things That Went Well

Resistance / Challenges

Cool-Down Notes

Homework / Drills for Next Time

Warm-Up

What did you do? How did the horse feel?

Focused Exercises

Flatwork Goals

_____

_____

_____

Breakthroughs / Things That Went Well

Resistance / Challenges

Cool-Down Notes

Homework / Drills for Next Time

Daily Schooling Session Log

Date: _____ Horse: _____   Date: _____ Horse: _____

Warm-Up

What did you do? How did the horse feel?

Warm-Up

What did you do? How did the horse feel?

Focused Exercises

Flatwork Goals

_____

_____

_____

Focused Exercises

Flatwork Goals

_____

_____

_____

Breakthroughs / Things That Went Well

Breakthroughs / Things That Went Well

Resistance / Challenges

Resistance / Challenges

Cool-Down Notes

Cool-Down Notes

Homework / Drills for Next Time

Homework / Drills for Next Time

Daily Schooling Session Log

Date: _____   Horse: _____   Date: _____   Horse: _____

Warm-Up

What did you do? How did the horse feel?

Warm-Up

What did you do? How did the horse feel?

Focused Exercises

Flatwork Goals

_____

_____

_____

Focused Exercises

Flatwork Goals

_____

_____

_____

Breakthroughs / Things That Went Well

Breakthroughs / Things That Went Well

Resistance / Challenges

Resistance / Challenges

Cool-Down Notes

Cool-Down Notes

Homework / Drills for Next Time

Homework / Drills for Next Time

Monthly Conditioning Check-In

Monthly Conditioning Check-In

Month: _____

Conditioning & Performance Progress

Circle or shade progress level for each category.

Quality	Needs Work	Improving	Strong
Fitness	○	○	○
Strength	○	○	○
Suppleness	○	○	○
Relaxation	○	○	○
Responsiveness to Aids	○	○	○
Rider Balance	○	○	○

Reflections

- What improved the most?

- What needs more focus next month?

- Any changes in tack, health, or schedule?

Monthly Conditioning Check-In

Month: _____

Conditioning & Performance Progress

Circle or shade progress level for each category.

Quality	Needs Work	Improving	Strong
Fitness	○	○	○
Strength	○	○	○
Suppleness	○	○	○
Relaxation	○	○	○
Responsiveness to Aids	○	○	○
Rider Balance	○	○	○

Reflections

- What improved the most?

- What needs more focus next month?

- Any changes in tack, health, or schedule?

Monthly Conditioning Check-In

Month: _____

Conditioning & Performance Progress

Circle or shade progress level for each category.

Quality	Needs Work	Improving	Strong
Fitness	○	○	○
Strength	○	○	○
Suppleness	○	○	○
Relaxation	○	○	○
Responsiveness to Aids	○	○	○
Rider Balance	○	○	○

Reflections

- What improved the most?

- What needs more focus next month?

- Any changes in tack, health, or schedule?

Monthly Conditioning Check-In

Month: _____

Conditioning & Performance Progress

Circle or shade progress level for each category.

Quality	Needs Work	Improving	Strong
Fitness	○	○	○
Strength	○	○	○
Suppleness	○	○	○
Relaxation	○	○	○
Responsiveness to Aids	○	○	○
Rider Balance	○	○	○

Reflections

- What improved the most?

- What needs more focus next month?

- Any changes in tack, health, or schedule?

Monthly Conditioning Check-In

Month: _____

Conditioning & Performance Progress

Circle or shade progress level for each category.

Quality	Needs Work	Improving	Strong
Fitness	○	○	○
Strength	○	○	○
Suppleness	○	○	○
Relaxation	○	○	○
Responsiveness to Aids	○	○	○
Rider Balance	○	○	○

Reflections

- What improved the most?

- What needs more focus next month?

- Any changes in tack, health, or schedule?

Monthly Conditioning Check-In

Month: _____

Conditioning & Performance Progress

Circle or shade progress level for each category.

Quality	Needs Work	Improving	Strong
Fitness	○	○	○
Strength	○	○	○
Suppleness	○	○	○
Relaxation	○	○	○
Responsiveness to Aids	○	○	○
Rider Balance	○	○	○

Reflections

- What improved the most?

- What needs more focus next month?

- Any changes in tack, health, or schedule?

Monthly Conditioning Check-In

Month: _____

Conditioning & Performance Progress

Circle or shade progress level for each category.

Quality	Needs Work	Improving	Strong
Fitness	○	○	○
Strength	○	○	○
Suppleness	○	○	○
Relaxation	○	○	○
Responsiveness to Aids	○	○	○
Rider Balance	○	○	○

Reflections

- What improved the most?

- What needs more focus next month?

- Any changes in tack, health, or schedule?

Monthly Conditioning Check-In

Month: _____

Conditioning & Performance Progress

Circle or shade progress level for each category.

Quality	Needs Work	Improving	Strong
Fitness	○	○	○
Strength	○	○	○
Suppleness	○	○	○
Relaxation	○	○	○
Responsiveness to Aids	○	○	○
Rider Balance	○	○	○

Reflections

- What improved the most?

- What needs more focus next month?

- Any changes in tack, health, or schedule?

Monthly Conditioning Check-In

Month: _____

Conditioning & Performance Progress

Circle or shade progress level for each category.

Quality	Needs Work	Improving	Strong
Fitness	○	○	○
Strength	○	○	○
Suppleness	○	○	○
Relaxation	○	○	○
Responsiveness to Aids	○	○	○
Rider Balance	○	○	○

Reflections

- What improved the most?

- What needs more focus next month?

- Any changes in tack, health, or schedule?

Monthly Conditioning Check-In

Month: _____

Conditioning & Performance Progress

Circle or shade progress level for each category.

Quality	Needs Work	Improving	Strong
Fitness	○	○	○
Strength	○	○	○
Suppleness	○	○	○
Relaxation	○	○	○
Responsiveness to Aids	○	○	○
Rider Balance	○	○	○

Reflections

- What improved the most?

- What needs more focus next month?

- Any changes in tack, health, or schedule?

Monthly Conditioning Check-In

Month: _____

Conditioning & Performance Progress

Circle or shade progress level for each category.

Quality	Needs Work	Improving	Strong
Fitness	○	○	○
Strength	○	○	○
Suppleness	○	○	○
Relaxation	○	○	○
Responsiveness to Aids	○	○	○
Rider Balance	○	○	○

Reflections

- What improved the most?

- What needs more focus next month?

- Any changes in tack, health, or schedule?

Monthly Conditioning Check-In

Month: _____

Conditioning & Performance Progress

Circle or shade progress level for each category.

Quality	Needs Work	Improving	Strong
Fitness	○	○	○
Strength	○	○	○
Suppleness	○	○	○
Relaxation	○	○	○
Responsiveness to Aids	○	○	○
Rider Balance	○	○	○

Reflections

- What improved the most?

- What needs more focus next month?

- Any changes in tack, health, or schedule?

Rider Awareness Scan

(USE BEFORE MOUNTING OR MID-RIDE.)

- ARE MY HANDS FOLLOWING, NOT HOLDING?
- ARE MY SHOULDERS SOFT?
- DO MY HIPS SWING FREELY WITH THE GAIT?
- AM I BREATHING LOW?
- IS MY ATTENTION ON THE HORSE, OR ON "GETTING IT RIGHT"
- RETURN TO ALIGNMENT → RHYTHM → BREATH

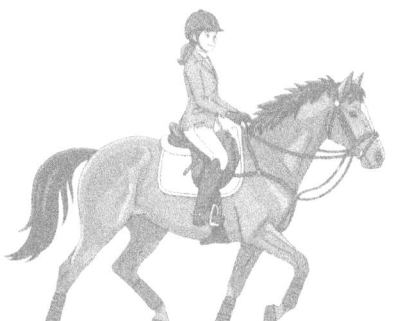

Troubleshooting Guide: When Things Don't Feel Right

What You Feel	Likely Cause	Simple Fix
Horse rushing	Tension or imbalance	Slow tempo with seat, not reins
Heavy in contact	Leaning vs lifting	Add transitions within gait
Drifting through shoulder	Lack of straightness	Add shoulder-fore
Losing forward	Unclear leg aid timing	Half-halt → ask → reward immediately

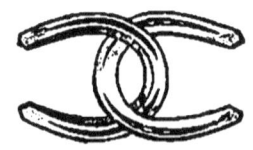

www.ingramcontent.com/pod-product-compliance
Lightning Source LLC
Chambersburg PA
CBHW052036070526
44584CB00016B/2067